A Choice Theory Guide to

STRESS

Ways of managing stress in your life

Brian Lennon

From "The Choice Theory in Action Series"

Copyright © 2019 Brian Lennon

All rights reserved.

ISBN: 9781097623976

Dedicated to
the memory of
Linda Harshman
whose serenity and humour
remain with us

CONTENTS

The Choice Theory In Action Series	vi
Acknowledgments	vii
Preface	ix
1. Stress and You	1
2. Choice Theory Psychology	13
3. The Choice Theory View of Stress	27
4. Choice Time	36
5. Identifying the Frustrations	44
6. Self Esteem	52
7. Relationships	59
8. Managing Your Time	70
9. Getting enough Sleep	79
10. Work	83
11. Checking Your Basic Needs	95
12. Decisions and Plans	103
13. Emergency Strategies	109
14. Getting Help	116
Further Reading	120
William Glasser International	122

The Choice Theory In Action Series

This is one of a series of short books aimed at helping people gain better control of their lives using ideas from Choice Theory psychology, a theory of human behaviour that was developed by Reality Therapy creator Dr. William Glasser.

In this selection of books we explain the application of Choice Theory psychology to a range of popular themes such as Addiction, Anger, Depression, Happiness, Parenting, Relationships and Stress. The authors are all experts in Choice Theory psychology and all have studied directly under its creator, Dr. William Glasser.

Hopefully this particular book will give you a brand new understanding of stress and practical ideas for dealing with it in your own life.

Brian Lennon
Series Editor

Acknowledgments

An American social reformer called Henry Ward Beecher once said, "How many a man has dated a new era in his life from the reading of a book!" Well, in my case it was not so much a book as a meeting back in 1985, an encounter that really did change so many things in my life.

My friend and colleague Arthur Dunne had invited me to a talk by Dr. William Glasser. At that time Glasser was known internationally for his "Reality Therapy", an approach to counselling he had created in the sixties. The introduction he gave in Dublin opened my mind to a host of new ways of understanding human behaviour and of intervening as a counsellor.

Just before the turn of the century Dr. Glasser formulated his "Choice Theory" and he introduced it as "a new psychology of personal freedom". This finally explained the theoretical base on which he had built and applied Reality Therapy. Since 1985 this understanding of human behaviour has been my guide both professionally and personally.

Dr. Glasser was my first teacher in this material and he was followed by a range of inspiring instructors and role-models: Suzy Hallock Bannigan, Richard Pulk, Al Katz, Don O'Donnell, Jim Montagnes and

Bob Wubbolding. Each of these has contributed in some way to the ideas that fill these pages and for that I am truly grateful. It has been my special good fortune to know Naomi Glasser, Carleen Glasser and Linda Harshman, three people who played enormous roles in Dr. Glasser's life and in ours.

Glasser's ideas fell on very fertile ground and I owe a great deal to the endless peer learning I have enjoyed in the company of Arthur Dunne, Jimmie Woods, Ken Lyons, Carmel Solon, Eileen Hearne, Sr. Claire Sweeney, Joan Meade, Marcella Finnerty, Sr. Basil Gaffney, John Brickell, Leon Lojk, Jagoda Tonsic-Krema and Juan Pablo Aljure. Indeed, I could fill many pages with the names of colleagues.

Arthur, Jimmie and Ken contributed some valuable comments on this book and I am especially grateful to them for that.

Finally, my constant inspiration and support is Laura and I can never thank her enough for being there, for her love and support.

Brian Lennon

Preface

For quite a number of years now I have been giving a presentation about Stress to teenagers here in Ireland. When first invited to do this I concentrated on the nature of stress itself and its plethora of unpleasant physiological changes.

Once I began to apply Choice Theory psychology to this topic it started to take on a different form. Stress was only the painful pointy edge of a deeper problem or problems. Soon I realised that it would be a mistake to focus on stress itself since it was more of a symptom than a cause. Make no mistake about it; stress is not a pleasant or healthy condition. If it is not given effective attention it can lead to physical and psychological harm. The important point is that "effective attention" must direct at the underlying causes of stress and not simply at the symptoms.

There is no universal cause of stress. It can vary from individual to individual although some problems are more characteristic of specific groups. The frustration that is generating stress can be due to not knowing what to do or not being able to do something. The one thing common to all these frustrations is that the stressed person's life is not going the way he or she wants it to go.

In these pages I hope to give an understanding of stress from the perspective of Choice Theory psychology and, by way of example, to show how this approach might be used with some typical human problems. I would hope that the reader will gain more than an insight into stress. Choice Theory psychology can point the way to taking more responsibility for one's own life and to gaining greater personal freedom as a result. Hopefully these ideas will help you achieve greater balance and happiness in your life.

1. Stress and You

One moment I was falling asleep and only a matter of minutes later I was experiencing the most stressful moment of my life! A late-night phone-call let us know that a family member was in danger from poor health. There was absolutely nothing I could do. I lay there with every fibre of my being in high tension. Briefly all the ideas that I had picked up over the years about stress flashed through my brain and, at the same time, the horrid realisation that they could do little for me.

All I and my wife could do was wait and hope. It was a long, long night with no sleep that I can remember. Next day we got more uptodate information and gradually the stress subsided. One thing that played a big part in this release was that we were putting together a plan that would help turn our relative's health around. The initial shock and related stress were converting into some form of positive action.

Life will inevitably bring those moments of sudden high stress, moments when there seems to be no control possible but even then, the only way out of the stress is to do something about its cause. That will be a major theme in this book.

Stress is breaking out all over the place. It's the epidemic of our age. It's almost reaching a point where people will worry if they are not worried about something. One of the very few good things we can say about stress is that at least it helps us feel we are part of some global movement but it is not a movement we want to belong to.

In spite of its epidemic-like status, stress is not some rare disease that afflicts a lot of human beings. In fact it is neither rare nor is it a disease. It is a very unpleasant psychological condition that almost everyone will experience at some time in their lives. To have stress does not mean you are mad or bad. It is a very normal human experience but it can seriously mess up your life and happiness.

Your body feels a constant tension and butterflies have a field day in the pit of your stomach. It's like a face-lift that affects your whole body. It's as if someone picked one part of your skin and tried to pull all the rest of your body covering into that one spot. Surface tension all over! It does not get any better at night. Eyes that cannot sleep and a brain that is full of ever increasing spirals of confusion! Then you wake up to greet the new day's challenges with a fabulously well-depleted set of batteries and flickering head-lights. It's no wonder the metaphors get mixed. That's not just stress in action; that's the story of your life and it's no laughing matter!

In fact, there is one positive aspect of stress, one it shares with both depression and anger. It is a sign that you have strong values. Something or someone matters to you and matters a great deal. Stress is the sign that this something or someone important to you is not as you would like it to be. If you didn't care about anyone or anything you would not experience stress at all. Stop giving a damn and all will be well! Take something to forget your woes and all will be grand! I hope you didn't believe that!

We can all experience brief periods of stress such as when we are running late for an important meeting or even when getting ready to declare our undying love to someone. These stress flare-ups tend to fade as soon as the critical moment has passed. Just watch people's smiling faces coming out of the dentist's. These short-lived stresses are usually bearable.

However, for some people, stress is a major characteristic of their lives. Every day seems to be stressful. It wears them down and makes normal life extremely difficult if not impossible. In fact life can become fairly rough for those around them too. Stress encourages moodiness and quick tempers as well as negative emotions that endanger relationships. It often drives friends away just when they are most needed.

Stress becomes like a painful straight-jacket gradually closing in around a person's life, holding the person in its grip, blocking out joy and with no solution in sight. If you have constant stress in your life, it is not good for you and it is time to take effective action to control it. It's time to start a plan for escaping from the grips of this straight-jacket. First of all, we need to take a closer look at the nature of stress.

What is Stress?

According to Choice Theory psychology all our behaviour is made up of four inseparable components and these provide a useful way to describe stress. The components are doing, thinking, feeling and physiology. Right now as you read these lines you are behaving and that behaviour is made up of doing, thinking, feeling and physiology.

Of course each person's experience of stress can vary a lot but here are some common experiences:

- Doing: some of us clench our teeth or fists, wrinkled forehead, generally tightened muscles.
- Thinking: we have dilemmas, conflicts, unresolved frustrations, not getting what we want.
- Feeling: trapped or severely restricted, overwhelmed, worn down.
- Physiology: tension in our muscles, aches and pains, palpitations, hyperventilation, increased blood pressure, headaches, digestive problems (even diarrhoea), sickness.

Stress could be defined in terms of a long list of unpleasant symptoms but at the heart of these are two main factors that generate all the symptoms:

- a serious frustration
- unresolved over time.

Billy has a struggle to bring in enough money to support his family and this has gone on for almost a year now. That is stress. Phil's total dedication to teaching and the long hours spent preparing class materials constantly contrasts with her principal's insistence on uniform checks in every class session. That is stress. It is a frustration, it's about something that matters and it lasts for some time, gradually wearing us down.

To deal effectively with stress it is not enough to focus on the symptoms; we need to address the long-standing unresolved frustrations and find ways of overcoming these.

An important thing to learn about stress is that it is not the real problem although admittedly it can become one in its own right. Stress is in fact part of our way of dealing with dangers or even the threat of danger. At the first signs of any problem we tend to become more alert and it is helpful to see how this state can develop into stress.

ALERT: Our senses sharpen and our eyes scan our surroundings, we prick up our ears. The bigger the threat the more we go on our own version of a "red alert".

ANXIETY: A basic state of alertness changes to anxiety if we see a situation that is somewhat out of our depth. That is what anxiety is telling us, "proceed with caution" … or even "stop and think!" Anxiety is the amber light of our psychological traffic system. Fear, a related experience, is the feeling that tells us we are facing something that is unknown. With anxiety we know what lies ahead and, at the same time, we know that we are not fully prepared for it.

Anxiety is actually an important feeling signal that is warning us to be careful, that we might not be fully prepared for what lies ahead. If things start to go seriously wrong that anxiety can spiral out of control to become panic. I am reminded of my car seat-belt! Forget to put it on and it begins to beep, a car-belt version of anxiety. Ignore this initial beep and the system goes crazy with extra volume and frequency, the belt alarm's version of panic.

STRESS: Ideally when we get a warning signal that something is wrong, we stop, think and come up with a solution. What happens when we cannot find a solution? It is when any anxiety or frustration lasts for some time without being sorted out that it becomes stress. Stress has to do with prolonged pressure, a pressure that gradually exhausts us. The only way to stop stress from lasting too long is to find out what is causing it and learn how to deal with that.

The Emergency Response

The next time you are at a football match keep a close eye on the goal-keeper nearest you. Students of animal behaviour could write pages about the antics of these human specimens when the ball is at the far end of the field. They pick imagined grains of dust out of their gloves, kick the heads of nearby dandelions in slow motion, chat with the umpires and make a study of the cloud formations. No doubt if you were to talk to them they could hold forth on philosophical topics too. That's while the ball is at the far end of the field.

Suddenly the action moves into mid-field and it's as if a totally different person were popped into the goal mouth. The keeper straightens up and bounces nervously from foot to foot, massive gloved palms reaching out to either side like a strange twitching butterfly. The closer the ball gets to the goal, the earlier stiffness converts into a head-to-toe jumpiness. It's the "red alert area" and the keeper is showing what we call the "emergency response". It is a heightened state of alertness that normally serves us very well.

Stress is part of our so-called "emergency response", a special preparation for danger that we share with all animals. Both our psychology and our physiology pay attention to the initial warning signals and they shift into a special state of readiness for danger. It makes perfect sense if we examine each of the changes in our bodies that are all part of stress.

Our lungs do their best to supply the extra oxygen by breathing faster. Our heart pumps harder to send extra oxygen to the brain. Our senses become sharper so that we see better, hear better and even our sense of smell gets sharper. This is our body's way of turning up the sensitivity to danger. Our digestive system stops and, at best, we experience butterflies in the stomach, at worst we have diarrhoea, our body's way of lightening the load in readiness for bigger dangers.

Our emergency response is in fact a very clever set of strategies aimed at increasing our readiness for danger. But, just like any alarm that goes on and on, the signal itself can be annoying and can end up generating even more confusion, frustration and exhaustion. Alarm systems are meant to be heeded quickly and not left running for very long. No matter how wonderful our alarm system is, it is rendered useless if we do not heed it. The same can be said for stress.

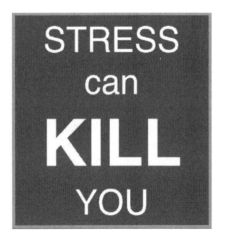

The build-up of the physical aspects of stress can be especially serious in people who already have health issues and medical support can be vital to these individuals. Whereas medication might have a role in alleviating the symptoms of stress in such people, it can never remove the problems that cause the stress in the first place.

The basic characteristics of stress eventually give rise to further problems: constant tiredness, poor sleep, diminished work productivity, weakened immune system resulting in many colds and infections, fibromyalgia, hypochondria, insecurity, period irregularities, loss of sexual drive, social withdrawal, irritability, personal neglect, comfort eating, loss of appetite. None of these is likely to be on anyone's bucket list! In short, a response that is designed to help us can become dangerous if it goes on too long. Like a fire alarm that just keeps ringing, it becomes a problem in itself.

Stress is Miserable

Even without the danger component, who wants stress? Prolonged unresolved stress is a miserable way to live a life. It's like carrying a heavy burden on our backs as we walk through life. Bowed under its pressure we fail to see a lot of the good things around us. It's hard to see the stars when you are bent over facing the ground. Stress is not kind to our natural good looks either, adding rashes and wrinkles, even premature ageing. No matter how useful stress is as a warning signal, we need stress like we need a hole in our heads. But it is not an illness; it's not something you inherited from your parents; it's not one of your national or racial traits. It is a very useful signalling mechanism but it becomes totally useless if you do not heed it.

Since I mentioned your parents, your race and nationality I had better clarify. It is true you might have learned some poor coping skills from any of these sources. You might also have inherited physical disadvantages that are difficult to cope with. You just might have more to deal with than other people but stress is the warning light. It is telling you that something needs fixing.

Buy a cheap pair of headphones and you are likely to get a manual translated into several world languages. No such luck for human beings. None of us was born with a book of instructions, about how to fix all the problems we encounter in life. Left to our own devices we tend to label stress as a problem in itself rather than as a symptom or signal of a problem and, if we think it is some sort of weakness or illness, we look for solutions in the wrong direction.

Attempted Solutions

Some of the solutions people find in books or online address the symptoms rather than the underlying causes. This is akin to recommending ear-plugs so as not to hear the fire alarm instead of suggesting how to put out the fire. At best these "solutions" can only be partially effective.

- Cutting back on work, study or responsibilities are not normally feasible options since the mere thought of doing this can increase the stress load especially if it means a reduction in income or status.

- Lying down and taking 20 deep breaths may give a few minute's relief at best and at worst leaves the individual still stressed but now breathless or dizzy.

- Imagining oneself lying on a beautiful beach with waves lapping gently under a cloudless sky challenges the stressed individual's imagination to the limits. For those with a good imagination such a fantasy might provide temporary escape but not a solution.

- A fantasy exercise such as blowing all the stresses into an imaginary balloon and letting it float away tends to be equally difficult and can challenge our credulity.

- Taking medication, alcohol or drugs that anaesthetise the brain and slow down the mind can also temporarily block out the stress only for it to return as an unwelcome visitor when the drug effects wear off. Worse still, prolonged use of these "remedies" can have serious physical consequences and the added stress of addiction. (Warning: Those currently taking psychiatric medication or any type of sedative should not stop without careful expert medical supervision.)

Admittedly some of these techniques might help some people but, at best, they can only alleviate the symptoms of stress since they make no attempt to address the underlying causes. Some familiarity with our own psychology is needed to help us understand how our behaviour works. Before examining some of the typical causes of stress and the corresponding remedies, we will explore Choice Theory psychology and what it might tell us about our stress.

2. Choice Theory Psychology

William Glasser was actually quite a shy individual when his book "Reality Therapy" surprised the psychiatric world in 1965. His ideas were already beginning to change the lives of many people who heard about them. This included one Fitzgeorge Peters in New York City. Fitzgeorge worked as a counsellor with victims of drug and alcohol addiction. Glasser's ideas were so meaningful to him that he upped camp, packed all his belongings into his Volvo car and headed west on a one-way trip to California to learn from Glasser himself.

As his knowledge of Reality Therapy grew, Fitzgeorge soon arrived at an interesting conclusion: "this is almost like a way of life". There was something about this new therapy that transcended the normal reach of psychotherapy. It was to be many years before Glasser himself twigged to the explanation, the fact that his therapy was based on a new understanding of human psychology.

That new understanding was Choice Theory psychology, an explanation of how and why we behave. Originally Glasser had looked for a theory that would explain what he did in Reality Therapy and Choice Theory was the answer.

Reality Therapy

Glasser's therapy was always based very much on the individual's control of his or her own life, on personal responsibility. Even today those who study this approach soon find that these ideas they learn in order to help others are actually a great help to themselves. Reality Therapy was not simply a set of techniques that a counsellor applied to clients, it provided a guide to personal well-being as well. In fact, counsellors cannot really help others with Reality Therapy unless they are already applying the ideas to their own lives.

The Origins of Choice Theory

In the nineteen eighties Glasser studied the writings of William Powers and Edwards Deming and these new ideas, combining with his basic understanding of Reality Therapy, led to the formulation of his new set of principles. I remember the excitement of those years as Glasser teased out the new ideas eventually adding his own to create "Choice Theory". In the book of that name published in 1998 Glasser called it a "new psychology of personal freedom". Choice Theory psychology was born! It was not simply an explanation of the processes of therapy but, as we shall see now, it also offered a more general explanation of human behaviour.

Who Is in Control of You?

At the heart of Choice Theory is the idea that the only behaviour you can control is your own. Not only that, but you control a lot more of your behaviour than you think. These core ideas of Choice Theory deserve a few hours' meditation. Can you think of anyone whom you really can control? For that matter, is there anyone who can control you? You might go along with what people want you to do sometimes but can they really control you?

The fact is that you cannot control others and they cannot control you. Unfortunately, that is not how most of us live our lives. Instead we think that we control each other. Each gender group jokes that it cannot control the other sex but then keeps trying to do so. We tend to work on the assumptions that we can control others and that others can control us. We blame others for our woes as if we were the hapless victims of their power over us. These assumptions can lead to all sorts of problems for us and they form the basis of what Glasser called external control psychology.

External Control Psychology

In our daily lives we tend to blame our problems on our inability to control others or on their apparent ability to control us. "I keep telling my son to tidy his room and he doesn't do it!" Somehow I think that I can really control my son. "The government drives me mad!"

Ah yes, it's the old story. The world would be a lot happier place if it didn't have other people in it! Wouldn't schools work better without pupils and hospitals without patients! Of course, the problem is not the people. The problem is when people try to control people! Glasser used to joke that the only real problem in life is that others will not do what we want them to do!

Without realising it we assume that others can control us and, conversely, that we can control them, two ideas doomed to failure. Glasser refers to this as the psychology of external control and it is the total opposite of his own internal control psychology, "Choice Theory". A life based on external control psychology will be a life of victimhood, misery and lots of stress. If we blame others for our misery we tend to wait for solutions to come from them and we could be a long time waiting. Although we tend to believe it is how the world works, this external control psychology is a major obstacle to our happiness.

Glasser offers a radically different psychology of human behaviour and a good starting point is to examine what he says about our needs.

Needs and Wants

Why are you reading this book, for example? Did someone force you to? Are you even reading the paragraphs in the order in which they were written? Even if you "had to" read this volume as part of a required reading list (heaven forbid), you still might opt not to read it or just to scan enough of it that you could pass an examination. In short, you are reading this because you chose to read it and, indeed, you are reading it the way you chose to read it. It might have been an almost unconscious choice but it was a choice and it was you who made it. So, the next question is, "why did you choose to read it?" I can only guess at your answers.

"I am reading it because I have nothing else to do (to pass the time)." "I am reading it because a friend recommended it." There can be lots of reasons ... because I have a stress problem ... because it might help a friend.

Glasser's explanation is that ultimately you are reading it in order to satisfy one or more basic needs. He identified five "Basic Needs" though he acknowledges that others may describe them differently.

Love and Belonging: our need to connect to people in friendly relationships. When I say, "I miss my friend", it is another way of saying that my love and belonging need is not being satisfied.

Power: the need to have some sense of control in our lives, to feel competent. Those who try to satisfy this as power over people place their belonging need in jeopardy. Glasser's view of power is about control of our own lives rather than control of others.

Freedom: the need to have sufficient space and time in our lives, space to be creative and to satisfy our needs without hindrance. We actually need not to be controlled by others.

Fun: a need that Glasser viewed as the genetic

reward for learning. As human beings we are constantly learning about new ways to enhance our lives and fun is the sparkle created by such new learning and new viewpoints.

Survival: the need to live, to be healthy, warm, safe and well-nourished. This is probably the most primitive of our needs.

Hopefully, by now, you will understand a little more about why you are reading this book. It could be to keep a friend happy (love and belonging), to increase your professional counselling skills (power), to get rid of some of the stress that has been dogging your life in recent times (freedom), to learn about a novel approach (fun) or to help reduce your increasing blood pressure (survival).

To read a book is not a basic need but it is a way of satisfying one or more basic needs. In fact each of us will have many ways of meeting our needs, ways we can classify as our "wants". It is these rather than the more theoretical "needs" that fill our waking hours as we work out how to realise them. It is our wants more than our needs that become the visible driving forces of our motivation.

Our Quality World

Glasser speaks of this collection of things we want as our "quality world", our personal repertoire of ways to meet our needs. Most human beings do not wander through life thinking about their basic needs. Instead they fill their heads with plans to achieve their wants. All our behavioural energy goes into making our wants happen but deep inside our personal psychology it is the needs that are ultimately seeking satisfaction.

Since our needs and wants are inside of us, Glasser then concludes that we control our own behaviour. We are not simply responding to external stimuli or rewards. It is the hunger inside of us that drives us.

If we ask, "why do we do what we do?" the Choice Theory answer would be that we are always trying to get what we want and we do that because we believe it will satisfy our needs. Even when someone else tells us what to do, we do what we ourselves want. When I obey someone else's orders it is because I have chosen to do so, because according to my own view of the world it makes better sense to obey that person than not to.

The "Quality World" is our world of wants. Right now I want a cup of coffee to take the chill out of the morning. Next week I want to go away with my family. I also want to see a television series a friend has recommended. All of these are wants. Some satisfy my need for survival, others my need for friendship and still others will meet my fun needs or a combination of needs.

Our "Quality World" is made up of people, situations, things, activities and even values that we work hard to achieve because we see them as need-satisfying to us. Other people's wants do not always make sense to us nor do ours to them. For one person a day spent fishing in a river is paradise but for another person, this would be a cold damp boring waste of time fiddling with hooks, lines and worms. Our wants might even include things that are illegal or harmful to ourselves and others. However, we choose them not because we think they will harm us but because we think they will be good for us. We think they will be need-fulfilling.

If you want a little rest from reading these pages, an interesting and often surprising exercise is to take a blank page and jot down a list of all the things, people, events that you yourself want right now. I do not mean all the things you might wish for but all that you really, really want, things you are striving to get or people you want to be with. If our wants play such an important part in our motivation, it makes sense to know what they are with some clarity!

Our Motivation is Internal

A deep philosophical question: why do you sometimes cross your legs? That might not be easy to answer but we could have better luck with a related question: did you choose to cross your legs? When I ask people this some of them stare at me as if I were accusing them of starting another world war and the others don that special look they display when questioning someone's sanity. Then, taking the question at face value, they look around to find someone they can "blame" for crossing their legs. Once they get over the initial shock of such a profound exploration of human behaviour they come to the realisation that they crossed their own legs; in fact, they actually chose to cross their legs.

The point here [...]
about choice. [...]
even aware of [...]
are still our cho[...]

Glasser believ[...]
behaviour. He [...]
goings-on such [...]
do indeed cho[...]
clear why we d[...]

choices we make that d[...]
not our survival.
Whatever choic[...]
more need-s[...]
choose th[...]
behavio[...]
stran[...]
co[...]

Why does a chi[...]
do people smok[...]
health risks associated with it? Why does someone
become obsessive about hand-washing? Why do
people cross their legs? Why do people answer
the telephone?

From a Choice Theory viewpoint all these people
are choosing behaviours that they believe to be
meeting their needs even when not conscious of
their choices. Let us go back to leg-crossing, for
example. You probably did not plan that in
advance. However, you cannot really say that
someone else crossed your legs; you did it. The
fact that you were not aware of it does not make it
any less your behaviour. This is important
because, if it was you who did it, it is you who can
undo it ... or even do it again. Once you realise
just how many choices you make, it becomes a
liberating idea since it means you could choose
something different.

As far as I know, nobody ever died because of
crossing their legs but there are many unconscious

...do threaten our happiness if...

...you make, if something else was ...atisfying in that moment you would ...at something else. Some of the ...rs people choose might strike us as ...e ways of meeting needs but when we ...sider their behaviour in depth we see how it ...orks.

For example, the smoker who knows clearly that this habit can cause cancer and other serious health problems continues to choose to smoke. It does not make sense! However, when you dig below the surface you may see that the person believes that stopping smoking would result in putting on weight (not necessarily true) and in being very grumpy for several weeks. The person also believes that smoking is relaxing (another myth). In other words, we can say that the smoker continues to smoke because he or she has more reasons for smoking than for stopping - even if these reasons are not all fully conscious or even accurate.

And so it is with all our behaviours. We choose them because we think they are good for us. That statement seems hard to accept if we consider behaviours such as stress or depression or even tiredness.

Total Behaviour

To understand why we sometimes choose behaviours that ultimately prove unpleasant for us we need to examine another key idea in Choice Theory, one we have already mentioned, that of "total behaviour".

If somebody were to ask you right now, "What are you doing?" you would probably say "reading". The fact is, you are "doing" a lot more than that. Hopefully all your bodily systems are chugging along nicely, your lungs taking in oxygen, your heart pumping the blood around your body and so on. Your mind is probably engaged in thought of some sort and your feelings world is hopefully one of calmness.

Glasser claims that our behaviour is not simply something we "do". In fact, it has four components and these four cannot be separated, hence the name "total behaviour". The components are "doing", "thinking", "feeling" and "physiology". By "physiology" we refer to all that goes on in the body, the circulation system, the breathing system, our immune system and the central nervous system. The doing, thinking, feeling and physiology are four components that all change together.

Have another look at your current behaviour, reading, and reflect on what is happening in each of the four components.

You suddenly remember you need to put the rubbish bins out on the road for collection! You abandon the book and struggle against the wind and rain outside, thinking you should really have gone to Spain when you had the chance, feeling miserable and your pulse is now a lot faster. From the point of view of personal choice this is interesting. You simply chose to put the bins out but, in doing so, you were choosing a completely different total behaviour.

When we choose a behaviour, we normally focus on something to do or something to think but, no matter which component we choose to change, all four components change together. If, for example, I sit down and start to recall a wonderful walk through the forest last week, my feelings and physiology begin to change in accord with my changes in doing and thinking. I begin to feel happy and my body relaxes. In Choice Theory terms I am actually choosing not only my doing and thinking but also my feeling and physiology. This is a very important point as it shows how we can manage our feelings and even our physiology.

The experience of stress is principally one of feeling bad and having unpleasant physiological changes but, according to Choice Theory psychology, it also involves doing and thinking. Once we change our doing or thinking, we also change our feeling and physiology. They all operate together. In fact, we can only change the feeling and physiology by changing the doing and/or the thinking. Change any one component and we change our total behaviour.

We will apply this to stress in more detail later but a brief example is in order here. When we are stressed we tend to focus mainly on what we feel and all the symptoms that show up in our physiology. Many of the books we read about stress focus on these and invite us to do breathing exercises and relaxation exercises, an emphasis on physiology. In Choice Theory, we prefer to focus on the thinking and doing. That is the major shift in emphasis that Choice Theory invites us to consider.

Something similar happens in how depression is interpreted. A major component is the loss of hope, not seeing any way to fix a situation. However, psychiatry tends to focus on an unproven physiological problem, a chemical imbalance. Fix the wrong cause and you get the wrong solution.

Somehow or other, we are choosing a total behaviour that includes these feelings and physiology. Once we realise this, then we find that making changes in our doing and thinking will bring about changes in these other signs of stress. That does not mean it will be easy but focusing exclusively on our feeling and physiology is very unlikely to remove our stress. The feelings are not free-floating; they have to do with very real frustrations in our life.

The Origins of Frustration

Watch a poor child in the midst of a tantrum and you are observing frustration in one of its purest forms. In Choice Theory we view frustration as the result of not getting what we want. In my mind's eye I have an idea of what I want (e.g., a satisfying job) but what I see in my life is very different (e.g., long hours, unfriendly colleagues, a tough boss and poor pay). The bigger the difference between what I have and what I want, the bigger the frustration.

Like the Rolling Stones, we "can't get no satisfaction". Frustrations are two-a-penny in most people's lives. All day every day we have a sequence of minor frustrations, many of which we barely notice. We fix them and get on with it. A button comes undone and we close it. We spill milk and we wipe it up ... except for those who choose to cry about it rather than fix it. The bus does not come on time. There is no milk for the coffee.

Sometimes, however, along comes a whopper of a frustration, where something very important is not working out as we want. At work I am expected to do 36 hours of work in a 24 hour day! My most important relationship is in the doldrums, or worse, is in the middle of a storm. My child is sick and the doctor thinks it might be serious.

Such major frustrations can become unbearable if we do not know what to do. We want to fix it but don't know how. If I do not realise I can make changes to my life or if I do not know how to make those changes, then the frustration can go on and on. That is what stress is all about, an important frustration that has gone on for too long ... or a lot of smaller frustrations that have outstayed their welcome!

3. The Choice Theory View of Stress

For many people "emotional intelligence" is a bit of an oxymoron, two words that seem to contradict each other. You either use your intelligence or you use your emotions, they would have us believe! "You are being emotional!" is a standard debater's ploy to curtail the opposition, a ploy that, paradoxically, could be called emotional blackmail!

In spite of the bad press our emotions have endured, there are signs of a change in attitudes towards them. Although psychologists sometimes argue about the differences between "emotions", "sentiments" and "feelings", there is a general acceptance nowadays that understanding one's feelings is a form of intelligence, a human skill worthy of developing. Choice Theory psychology has always given great importance to feelings and spells out a very specific role for them.

For William Glasser, feelings are centre-stage in human psychology. He once wrote that, "it is the hope of feeling good or better, immediately or later, that drives all of our behaviour." If our needs are the ultimate goal of our behaviour and our wants (quality world pictures) are the more tangible targets we aim for, the feelings are the barometer of our success in achieving these.

It is for this very reason that a Reality Therapy counselling session will rarely start with a question about the client's feelings. Glasser used to joke that such a question was superfluous since counselling clients were usually quite miserable when they arrived. As the counselling progresses, the Reality Therapy practitioner pays huge attention to the client's feelings and we are about to explore the reasons for this.

Indeed, to reach a fuller understanding of stress as viewed by Choice Theory psychology we need to learn more about this special importance it gives to feelings.

Feelings are Signals

We have already seen that Choice Theory acknowledges feeling as one of the four components of Total Behaviour. Elaborating on feelings Choice Theory claims they are signals.

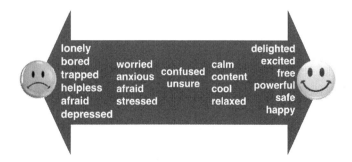

Their main task is to let us know how well we are running our lives. Specifically they tell us how well we are meeting our needs. We feel good when our needs are being met and bad when they are not. More specific feelings give us more specific information about our needs.

For example, neglect your belonging needs and you will feel lonely. Disregard your health and you will feel unwell. When your freedom need is not being fed you feel trapped. Forget about your fun need and you will feel bored. When your power need is neglected you feel weak or helpless. When any needs are not being well met you can feel sad, bad or low. When the need batteries are running close to empty and you don't know what to do about it you feel depressed.

At the other end of the scale feelings such as happiness, joy, freedom, confidence, excitement, healthy are all indicators of needs being met.

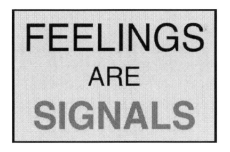

The Feeling of Frustration

In Choice Theory psychology we believe that frustrations arise because of the discrepancy we see between what we have and what we want. I want €100 to buy a gift for my partner but I only have €20. I am frustrated to the tune of €80! In Choice Theory language there is a difference between my perceived world (€20) and my quality world (€100). The bigger that difference, the bigger my frustration.

Frustration is that special feeling that points to the distance between what I want and what I have got! In frustration we feel the pain of the gap in our lives. In Ireland we have a special talent for describing this feeling. We will say, "I went to the car park and there was my car, stolen". Again, in the Irish language, to say "I miss you" we have "mothaím uam thú" which translates literally as "I feel you away from me".

Signals for Action

Once you accept the notion of feelings as signals then it becomes harder to ignore them or to misconstrue them. Of course, if I label some of my feelings as "illnesses" or even as weaknesses that I have inherited from my parents, I am unlikely to do very much about them except perhaps, seek some sort of psychological pain-killer!

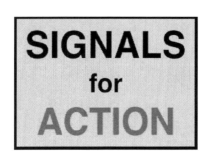

But feelings are neither illnesses, defects nor disorders. Instead they are very important parts of our psychology and we do well to heed them. Signals don't exist in a vacuum. On the one hand they have a cause and, on the other, they have a purpose and that purpose is action.

This is equally true about physical feelings. If something I touch with my finger feels very hot, a fast signal goes to my brain and I rapidly pull my finger back from the heat. In fact, if we could not feel pain we would be in serious danger of harming ourselves regularly.

It is interesting that we seem to have learned how to deal with physical pain but not with psychological pain. When I accidentally sit on a hot stove, I do not sit there with part of my anatomy cooking and waiting for someone to rescue me. The alarm bells in my head instruct me to hop up quickly. When I get similar alarms about psychological pain, society would have me believe that I have an illness, something that can only be treated (since no cure is ever guaranteed) by outside intervention. With such thoughts I continue to sit it out on my psychological hot stove while my soul is sizzling away!

When we feel miserable we sometimes moan and grumble, blaming others or our genes or the weather or some as-yet undiscovered chemical imbalance. Choice Theory takes a different approach and recommends us to take our feelings seriously for what they are, signals for action. A painful feeling is telling you something is wrong and invites you to fix it. Stress is no different.

Stress is a Signal

So what is the stress feeling telling us? Well, it is certainly shouting out that something is wrong. The mistake is to think that stress is the problem. That would be like blaming the fire alarm for the fire.

Thinking that stress is like some sort of illness that has invaded our bodies is a variant of external control psychology, the idea that we are controlled from the outside. Stress, far from being an invader, is a vital part of our internal alarm system. If we believe that stress is an illness or even if we focus excessively on the external factors contributing to our stress we are unlikely to adopt an approach that will be effective in reducing our stress,

However painful stress might seem to us it is simply a signal that is telling us that we are not meeting our needs well. In practice this usually means that there is something we want that we are not getting or that something is not the way we want it to be.

The big difference between feeling stress and merely feeling bad or frustrated is that stress has an important time component. It is a feeling of frustration that has lasted for some time. Frustration is unpleasant in itself but if it goes on and on it becomes the even more unpleasant experience that is stress.

Unless we heed our signals and then address the root causes of our stress, minimising the symptoms will be counter-productive. When a fire alarm sounds we do not go seeking an electrician to snip the wires and stop the annoying sound. Instead we heed the signal and extinguish the fire that triggered it. Whether we try to silence our stress signals with relaxation exercises or with any type of drug, the stress will continue unless we address its root cause.

Stress is a set of feelings and physiological changes that arise from prolonged frustration of our basic needs. As such, stress is a red alert, telling us that something is amiss. We need to focus our attention on identifying and fixing the underlying frustration.

Anxiety is a Signal

Anxiety is another signal and it is important to understand its message. Anxiety warns us that somehow we are facing a situation that we are not fully equipped to deal with. It is a very useful signal that tells us we are getting out of our depth. A big difference between anxiety and stress is that stress has a longer life. The frustration has lasted longer and this suggests that the individual has been unable to seek or find solutions to that frustration. Indeed the person might not even be fully aware of being frustrated and, even if aware, might not have a clue as to what the cause is. Of course, if our anxiety lasts for a long time it becomes stress.

Panic can set in when anxiety escalates out of control. Those who have not developed the habit of taking action on the earlier feeling signals of anxiety are destined to have the alarm bells increase in volume. Panic or stress that is not dealt with will gradually wear a person down and may give rise to serious health problems.

Fear is a Signal

Fear too is telling us something. If anxiety is about something we know but are not sufficiently prepared for, fear is about the unknown and so it is impossible to prepare for it. The message is clear: don't go there! The solution for fear is knowledge; find out more about the cause of our fear. As always in Choice Theory, feelings are signals and are calling out for active intervention.

Bringing It All Together

Now we can summarise what Choice Theory psychology teaches us about dealing with stress and in subsequent chapters we will look at some of these steps.

1. Recognise stress as an internal alarm, not as a disease or weakness.
2. Consider stress as a feeling telling us things are not working for us.
3. It is informing me that I am not getting what I want.
4. It is also telling me to do something about it!
5. Set aside time to deal with my stress.

6. Examine my current life to identify the major frustrations.
7. If I cannot identify the cause of my stress I should get help in doing this.
8. Learn any new skills or ideas that are required to make the changes.
9. Make changes to what I want or to what I am doing to get it.
10. Review my progress and make any necessary changes or adjustments.

The first few steps above are dealt with in the earlier chapters of this book. Step five, taking time to deal with your stress, is one that only you, the reader, can take. Reading this book is part of that but it is important to stop and take the time to apply the ideas to your own life. In fact, time for reflection is so important that I intend doing that right now, creating a special chapter about the topic.

4. Choice Time

As children we had a wonderful little "magic" trick we would play on unsuspecting friends. As a firm believer that some part of childhood should be kept forever, I must confess to playing this same trick now and again even today. You yourself can even have a go right now. Follow these three simple instructions before you read any further.

1. Stand near a wall with your arm outstretched so that your fingers just tip the wall.
2. Then lower your arm and rub that elbow about five times with your other hand.
3. Now, no matter how hard you try, your finger tips will no longer reach the wall!

Of course, the "magic" has nothing to do with the elbow at all but has everything to do with the instructions about "no matter how hard you try". This wording suggests that you should try hard and this trying converts into a straining of the muscles which in turn shortens them. The end result is that the attempt to stretch the arm actually shortens it, a paradox.

The Paradox of Stress

A similar paradoxical dynamic can mean that stress easily becomes self-perpetuating. We get into a rut that generates our stress. For some strange reason we tend to conclude that staying in the rut is necessary even seeing it as the way to get rid of our stress! We strain our psychological muscles! We become obsessive and stick our nose even closer to the grind-stone that is wearing us down.

The reason for this bizarre behaviour is that stress is not conducive to creative thinking or learning. When things are not going well and we experience stress, our capacity to consider solutions is severely hampered by that very stress. We develop cognitive short-sightedness and tunnel vision!

It makes sense! When I am under attack my whole mental processing goes into defence mode; I want to survive. My entire focus is now on a branch to grab hold of, a life ring to use, a quick solution, any solution. Stress, like any danger signal, induces a sense of urgency but, in most cases, this urgency is more imagined than real.

What we need to do is to pre-program our heads with a simple thought: when we get red warning lights, it's time to stop and think. In other words, stop at the lights! What we need is what I am calling "Choice Time". There is a saying that is popular in the United States: "Keep doing what you are doing and you will keep getting what you have got!" It makes sense, therefore, to stop doing what we are doing. Just stop. Make the choice to put on the brakes.

Even if it's not a full "stop-and-think" break, just

stopping for a while would be an improvement. This in itself is not going to solve your stress problem but it is a necessary first step. You cannot examine your problems and consider solutions without stopping to reflect.

There is a devious little voice in our heads that continually tries to trick us into disaster. This little demon tells us that we don't have the time to stop. When we are in a hurry to get to our destination by car, it's that same demon that insists that we don't have time to stop for petrol. Fortunately a second saner voice reminds us that we are not going to reach our destination without re-fuelling, something that is hard to do without stopping.

The demon voice has a field day with stress and plants a series of dangerous ideas: "I cannot stop working so hard or my stress will increase!" "Talking to my partner will probably make things worse!" "I don't have the time to take a break!"

At these times we badly need to listen to the other voice, the sane voice. Give it the chance and it will remind you that stopping for petrol makes sense and that having a rest break from work makes the same sense. It will explain that letting stress or even tiredness accumulate is not a good idea. It will even help you understand how the demon voice takes advantage of your sense of urgency to lead you astray.

Choice Theory very much aligns itself with the sane voice. It recommends taking responsibility for what is happening in your life. The first step is to put your foot on the brake, just stop. Later we will look at a fuller version of this Choice Time break but, for now, we look at different ways to stop.

Pause

Doing anything for long periods of time without a break is not a good idea. Try holding your arm out to your side for as little as sixty seconds and you will see what I mean. Just stop and do something different for five minutes. You might want to try it now. Just go and have a coffee or a short walk around the house or garden.

Stress, after all, is prolonged pressure; it is pressure plus time. Breaking up that time is a wonderful first defence against the build-up of pressure we call stress. If you really like stress, just cancel your breaks!

People who work or study without breaks do not do themselves favours since both work and study suffer. More important is that the individual suffers with risks for health and fitness.

Do Something Different

Both our minds and bodies benefit from change. Sitting or standing in the same posture for too long can tire our bodies. Something similar happens in our minds when we focus on the same subject matter for too long.

Having a break is important and the more different that is from our original behaviour the better.

Coffee and lunch breaks in work places are very important since they are a change from the work itself. People return to work with more energy and refreshed minds. Not only do the workers feel better but they also perform better and productivity, paradoxically, improves if there are adequate breaks.

Seamus is a good friend of mine and, when he was a student, he used to work in a furniture factory in the summer months. As a good organiser his talents were soon recognised and he was placed in charge of the summer workers. He drew the boss's attention to the fact that his employees did not have a morning break. The boss was reluctant to change as he feared that productivity would suffer too much. Seamus is an Ulster-man and we do not give up easily! He asked if he could try a 15-minute break every day for a fortnight. The boss agreed. When figures were reviewed two weeks later, productivity had increased by 25%.

Move About

In our increasingly sedentary world we need to become more deliberate about building movement into our lives. Taking a break by having a cup of coffee on the same chair we use for our work is an odd version of a break!

Staying still for too long is not good for circulation or general physical well-being. Build movement into your work if you can and certainly make it part of your break. Stretch arms and legs, move around, go for a walk or swim.

Apart from shorter breaks during our working hours, it is important to ensure we have adequate exercise every day. Even 30 minutes walking will enhance our overall health prospects. However, don't take your stress with you. Enjoy the walk, rejoice in the scenery, have a chat with a friend, throw the ball for the dog, anything but stressful thoughts and conversation.

This is not to say you forget about your stress. Quite the opposite! Select a time and place to deal with it. Take it seriously, very seriously. But take your breaks just as seriously since they will contribute to your overall success.

Get Water and Air

A clear head requires oxygen and water! Ventilate your work area well and always have drinking water nearby. Both body and mind require these two commodities for successful functioning.

The Ideal Break

So, join all the above items into one and you have the ideal break: a total change with movement, air and water! Some of the most successful businesses in the world are now creating special recreational areas within the work place where employees can go to unwind, play music, do exercises in a gym, draw and paint ... have a break!

Having breaks, not only at work but also in our home lives, is one of the best ways to avoid stress because it breaks the accumulation effect. When stress has built up in our lives we need a more focused break, one I think of as "the full version".

Choice Time, the Full Version

When we are experiencing stress we need to set aside special time to address the frustration with all the seriousness that it deserves. Stress is a huge alarm signal and points to a big frustration, one that merits our full attention. A red alert is not much good if the emergency services do not respond.

The simple logic is this: if we do not set aside time to tackle our stress we will not be able to tackle our stress! You cannot mend a puncture while the car is still moving. It's a good idea to begin this process by planning a short break to focus on stress, one that allows you sufficient time to make a preliminary list of your frustrations and that becomes the topic for our next chapter.

Right now you can have a peek at your busy calendar and choose a time to start dealing with your stress. Keep the time short (maybe 15 minutes) so that you have a good chance of actually keeping to your plan. It is unnecessary and unwise to attempt to plan the rest of your life at this point. A simple fifteen minute session will probably be more than adequate to start the process.

Later chapters will offer some suggestions for dealing with specific areas of difficulty but first we need to identify our problem areas.

5. Identifying the Frustrations

So stress is the red traffic light telling us to stop whatever we have been doing because something is not the way we want it to be. The next step is to pinpoint what exactly is generating the frustration signals. This calls for a full serious "Choice Time" break to take a long hard look at our lives.

Remember, stress is not the problem; stress is the end-result of the problems you have. Having problems and knowing we have them can be two very different things. Similarly, knowing what the problem is and knowing how to fix it can be equally different.

First, it may help to examine some typical frustration areas, experiences that can touch the lives of almost anyone. There are other issues that are more likely to appear at a particular age or in a particular group of people.

The following lists are by no means exhaustive nor are they divided in a rigid way. Their main purpose is to help you see that stress can be broken down into specific problem areas in your life. Stress is not some strange affliction that descends upon us from the unknown. It is a really good alarm system but a total nuisance if we ignore it or do not know what action to take. You don't fix stress directly; you fix the problems that have generated the stress. When the oil warning light comes on in your car, you fix the oil problem not the light problem! We need to learn to treat our bodies and minds at least as well as we treat our cars.

Common Problems

No matter who we are or how much experience or education we have, there will always areas of life that we know little about. These are the areas that are most likely to create stress in our lives. None of us are born knowing everything nor with a guide book to life tied to our legs!

Here are some common areas of difficulty that people experience.

- I have problems in a relationship that is important to me.
- I find it hard to mix with people.
- I have very little self-confidence, low self-esteem.
- I am not good at planning.
- I am studying for examinations but I do not seem to be learning enough.
- I have concerns about my health.
- I am looking after someone and it is proving very difficult.
- I have worries about money.
- I am being bullied or teased.
- I seem to be addicted to something.
- I am not sleeping very well.
- I am not having enough fun in my life.
- I never seem to do anything right, no good luck.

- I sometimes get thoughts that scare me.
- Something terrible happened to me and I do not know what to do.

Problems of Youth

- I do not know how to relate to other people.
- I find it hard to deal with the opposite sex.
- I have doubts about my gender identity.
- I have constant problems with my parents.
- I am being bullied.
- I am very shy, find it hard to deal with social occasions.
- I find school and study very difficult.
- I am worried about my future.

Problems of Young Adults

- I cannot find a job.
- I have difficulty making ends meet.
- My relationships are not working well.
- I am having bad experiences on the social networks.
- I am drinking too much.
- I have problems at work.
- I have problems with mortgages.

Problems of Mid-Life

- I cannot keep up with the demands of my work-place.
- My boss or work-colleagues are proving difficult.
- I have constant rows with my teenage children.
- I am having problems with my partner.
- I have difficult caring responsibilities.

Problems of Later Years

- I have health concerns.
- I cannot face retirement.
- I do not have adequate plans for retirement.
- I find it hard to be retired.
- I worry about my health.
- I have many regrets.
- I often feel lonely.
- I sometimes feel very insecure.

Depression and Anxiety

Notice that these lists do not mention problems such as depression, anxiety, sadness, unhappiness. The reason for this apparent omission is that Choice Theory sees these "problems" as the signals of underlying frustrations. It is the underlying frustration that we need to deal with rather than the resulting feelings or physiology. This is a vital distinction since our attitude to this will determine how we deal with our problems.

It would be beyond the scope of this book to deal with every possible human problem. By taking a small selection of these later we hope to show how a Choice Theory approach might be used and that will help the reader apply these ideas to other situations that may arise. The first step is the most important, recognising stress as a signal that something needs to be fixed in our lives.

What is important is to take the time now to identify one or more areas of your life that are not working well. Some may be glaringly obvious to you (e.g., a shortage of money) but others may not be quite so apparent (e.g., not having enough fun). If you find it very difficult to identify the root causes of your stress then you are strongly recommended to consult with a friend or counsellor.

Overwhelm

This is a problem that rarely gets a mention and yet I have seen lots of people experience it. They find it hard to pinpoint any one cause of their stress and the reason is that in their case there is not simply one cause; there are lots of causes. A host of little things go wrong or they run out of the time needed to fix them. The day seems too short to manage everything.

They experience what used to be called "free-floating anxiety", a sinking feeling in the pit of the stomach that does not seem to have an explanation. I believe the reason is that they cannot see the forest for the trees, or even the leaves! There are so many relatively "little" things not working properly that they fail to identify them as problems and just get a general sense of life as doomed to misery and stress. The unfathomable is unfixable!

Increasing stress, like any alarm system, brings increasing confusion and the ability to identify and fix problems diminishes when we need it most.

The only way out of such a situation is to start somewhere. Pick one thing that you can change and go for it. Do not worry about the mountain that you still have to climb; worry about the first gate in your path. Overwhelm can easily induce a state of psychological paralysis, doing nothing instead of beginning somewhere.

This is a good example of the importance of "Choice Time", of stopping and reflecting. Call off the whirlwind for a little while, by all means take a few good breaths and then think about it. Focus on one reasonably accessible problem that you can begin working on straight away. Without a start there can be no finish … and you can only start from here.

Unhelpful Thoughts

Sometimes we are our own worst enemy. We spend time blaming ourselves instead of devoting that same time to thinking about change. We think, "I am no good at making friends" or "I am a useless parent" instead of "I am going to learn about how to make friends" or "I am going to improve my parenting skills". We may even blame our personal history. "Depression is in my genes." A belief in our own internal control is very important. No matter what complication I have in life I can choose to spend my time bemoaning my predicament or I can choose to begin the process of improving the situation. I have a choice between moaning and fixing. I have a choice.

Another unhelpful thought is to blame others for our stresses. It may very well be a fact that others play a big part in complicating our lives and contributing to our misery. However, the only person I can control is myself and so the first step in solving my problem will be my own choice to do something about it. This may in fact mean initiating discussion with the other person or persons but it will be my first step, my own choice that starts the process. No matter what I believe to be the origins of my current distress, that vital first step towards resolving it is my own.

The tendency to blame others or to moan about our miseries seems to be well-established in most of us. One way to keep all our devious psychological addictions happy is to set a limit. "I will moan about this for one hour and then I will start to fix it." Even in this we have a choice.

Where to Start

If you have quite a number of frustrations to work out then you may need to consider which one to start with and how to approach it.

Do not try and solve everything at once. It is usually a good idea to choose one area to begin with. Ideally this should be the least complicated. Then get ideas on how to change your approach to this area and, finally, plan small changes that are highly likely to be successful.

You could even try this right now. Identify one small problem you could fix in five minutes. Then decide whether or not you will fix it. This might not seem important but getting the momentum for change going is vital.

A Template for Change

1. What is the major problem for me, the issue that I tend to be thinking about when I experience the strongest feelings of stress? (I might need help in identifying this.)
2. How do I want things to be? Give specific details.
3. What have I tried so far as my best attempt to deal with this?
4. Have my attempts so far worked, have they got me what I want?
5. Do I need to change my approach, what I want or what I am doing to get it?
6. Do I know how to change? (I might need help in this.)
7. What am I going to start with?
8. What exactly am I going to do? (What? When? Where? How?)
9. When will I review progress and make adjustments?

The following chapters deal with examples of typical problem areas that many people encounter.

6. Self Esteem

We live in a world of "selfies". The fact is that we have always lived in a world of selfies. Long before the smart phone put a double-edged camera in our hands, we have been taking psychological pictures of ourselves. Gradually from some time in early adolescence each of us builds up a composite internal picture of ourselves. This "self-concept" works just like any other concept in our heads. If I perceive a particular chair to be uncomfortable then I will probably choose not to sit on it. How I perceive and, especially, how I value my "self" will determine what I choose to do with and about myself.

Whatever view we have of ourselves, it is one that accompanies us day and night. We cannot escape it and , if my self-esteem is low, it's like being stuck in a small space with someone I don't like! Low self-esteem has its own insidious way of contributing to stress.

Self Concept

Although psychologists sometimes differ about how to define "self-concept" it is essentially the view I have of myself; it's how I see myself. When we think of other people, we generally think of their personality or character. These are external observations of people and others will certainly have opinions about our own personality. How others see me is my "personality" but how I see myself is my "self-concept". It is my view of me!

I may see myself as intelligent, tall, deep thinking, friendly, Irish, interested in Art, lazy, having dandruff, and so on. Any of us could probably fill several pages with a self-description. However, some of these attributes will be more important to us than others. I might not care whether I am tall or short but the fat-slim dimension may be an obsession for me. In other words, some of the scales I use to evaluate myself will be more important to me than others.

In Choice Theory psychology, like several other psychologies, we believe that our perceptions of the world are important. We do not really behave according to the real world out there but according to our perceptions of it.

Many years ago I nipped into a wonderful little self-service cafeteria downtown Drogheda to have some lunch. After picking up a sandwich I noticed a very appetising apple tart so I added that to my tray. Nearby was a little jug of custard so I poured some over the apple tart. When I sat down I realised that the "custard" was in fact mayonnaise. I had behaved according to my perceptions and my perceptions were wrong! (The manager promptly gave me another dessert and hinted he might give mine to his staff!)

It's just the same with the concept I have of myself.

I behave according to that. If I label myself as a "bad student", I may avoid anything that looks like a course of study. Labels are dangerous. So many people emerge from years of education with probably inaccurate perceptions of themselves such as "bad at languages", "disastrous at mathematics", "not good at creative writing", "hopeless at art".

It makes good sense to challenge all these perceptions we have of ourselves. If there is something you like, go for it and do not worry too much about your perceived aptitude for it. There is no rule that says you should only do things you are good at! "Jack of all trades and master of none" is a horrible saying I threw out of my head a long time ago as it hampers self-development.

What is probably more important than the concepts I have of myself is the value I place on these and that leads into "self-esteem", the evaluative dimension of the self-concept.

The Value I have of Myself

Self-esteem is my evaluation of myself. It is not the evaluation others have of me nor the evaluation I have of others. If I place a dismal value on myself I will be in a continuous state of frustration. No matter where I am, no matter what I need to do, my poor dismal self will be there I will constantly regard myself as inadequate for whatever I need to do.

If Choice Theory psychology sees frustrations as signals of the discrepancy between what I have and what I want, then this low evaluation of self is a particularly important frustration, one we might call the "self-frustration". It is, of course, more commonly known as "low self-esteem". When the distance between how I see myself and how I want to see myself is large, I am experiencing low self-esteem.

Although we speak of self-esteem as if it were one single variable, it can be very complex. My overall evaluation of myself may depend on a number of internal scales based on the values I hold most dear. If a young man wants to be a good student, to excel on the rugby field and to be an expert in the Rubik cube, then his self-esteem will depend greatly on how he rates himself on these scales. My self-esteem is not simply my measure of me; it is my measure based on my own personal scales of measurement. I may rate very well in your eyes, in your scales of measurement but it is my own internal scales that matter as far as my self-esteem is concerned.

Self-loathing

Some people see so many differences between how they are and how they want to be that they end up hating themselves. They see themselves as hopeless cases, unlikeable by others and doomed to failure. The famous quotation attributed to Groucho Marx is very close to how many low self-esteem people think: "I don't want to belong to any club that will accept people like me as a member." If I have a very low opinion of myself and somebody is friendly to me, I begin to think they have ulterior motives; they could not possibly be friendly to me because they like me. It becomes a very complicated and a very sad world.

Low self-esteem means that the person will be in an almost permanent state of frustration and that's just another way of saying continuous stress. Social situations can be painful experiences. New relationships can be frightening. After all, won't that other person abandon me when she finds out what I am really like?

Friendly Advice

Low self-esteem people are often very caring towards others and are very sensitive to the needs of others. These qualities mean that they usually do have good friends who care for them. However, that does not mean that the advice offered by the friends is always helpful. Pals often shower the low self-esteem person with lots of praise: "But you are good-looking … and intelligent … and generous!" The problem is that the low self-esteem person does not believe these well-intentioned words. Not only that but they see a hidden message in the comments: "Not only do you have a low opinion of yourself but you are also wrong!"

So, what can a person do if experiencing low self-esteem? To understand this we need to recall how Choice Theory psychology interprets feelings.

Self-Esteem as a Signal

In Choice Theory all feelings of frustration are

signals and, as such, they are signals for action. Self-esteem is no different. My low self-esteem is a signal telling me that I am not happy with one or more important aspects of myself and, therefore, I should be doing something about it. It is a call to action not to self-pity.

In a sense I am saying that when you have a low opinion of yourself, you might be right! You are not the way you want to be and you are entitled to feel bad about that. Now, what are you going to do about it? You can choose to bemoan your unhappy state or you can begin to work on a plan for "self renovation".

I might think that I am far too overweight for my own good. In reality I might be the perfect weight for my height, age and gender. That does not matter. My view of myself is what matters to me. If I think I am the wrong weight, then, to all intents and purposes I am the wrong weight. I will behave as if I were overweight and I will continue to fret about it. So, what can I do?

Heeding the Signals

It makes sense for the low self-esteem sufferer to do some reality checking. If I think I am overweight, how could I verify this? I might consult with a doctor or dietitian about it, for example.

What is important is that I heed the frustration signals embedded in my low self-esteem. I do something about this inner tension between what I see and what I want to see. Once I clarify what my ideal weight should be I might plan a sensible diet to achieve this.

In other words, my low self-esteem is telling me (1) I am not happy with myself and (2) to do something to change myself so that I will become more happy with myself. It is important to make plans and to start with small highly possible steps. Become the sort of person you want to be instead of bemoaning your shortcomings. Convert stress and anxiety into proactive plans to improve yourself.

This is easy to say but difficult to do. The alternative is to do nothing and to continue to suffer all the secondary effects of low self-esteem. One thing worse that being criticised is to carry that critic around with you on a daily basis!

7. Relationships

In a scene reminiscent of the "Third Man" film, a gentleman in a trench coat walks along a sombre damp city street. He stops close to a dim street lamp, looks around and then cups his hands around his mouth to light a cigarette. A deep consoling voice from the technical stratosphere tells us that we are never alone with this cigarette. It was 1959 and the subject of this television advertising campaign never made it to the sixties. Nobody wanted a lonely dark damp street even with this magical cigarette and voice from above. In particular, it appeared that nobody wanted to be so alone as this bloke in the trench coat.

The vast majority of people want relationships of some sort. One way or another, relationships play an important part in our lives. If you look through your phone records at all the calls you made over the last week you will see the variety of your human contacts ranging from warm friendships to cooler business exchanges to practically anonymous calls, all some form of relationship. Your real-life contacts with others probably follow a similar spread.

There must be dozens of ways of classifying our relationships and one that will serve our purpose here would be a scale based on degrees of friendship: close friends, friends, acquaintances, unknowns, unfriendly, hostile.

Generally, we do not have major problems with those we consider as friends nor do we have many issues with those we gladly avoid or ignore. Where difficulties arise is with the people we have not fully chosen and whom we cannot easily avoid. This would apply to groups such as family, work colleagues and neighbours. We are born into these groups or are tied to them for reasons of career or physical proximity.

Glasser had a simple rule-of-thumb to help us relate to others. He recommended that we avoid using external control. In fact, the way we treat our friends is a good model of this, of using Choice Theory instead of external control. He wrote that, "we don't use external control with our very good long-term friends". Elsewhere he commented, "long-term friendships are the only human relationships where, without knowing what we are doing, we use choice theory from the start."

We normally do not try to control those we truly regard as our friends but sometimes we appear to get confused and use external control with people who are close to us and whom we want to stay close to.

Partners

One special type of friend is the "partner" ("spouse", "husband", "wife", "boy-friend" or "girl-friend"). Unlike the good friend we see from time to time, once we identify someone as a partner, we tend to share our lives with that person and that is where the difficulty arises. The partner soon qualifies for membership of a special category that borders on the "family" group, people we cannot really avoid.

So what is the potential source of stress in such relationships? According to Choice Theory it is the use of external control psychology. When I act in a way that suggests I am trying to control the other person, then the relationship can be damaged. A true friend does not try to control you and you do not try to control a true friend. Live with that friend for a while, however, and there is an increasing temptation to exercise control over the other.

For some reason the "partner" group has its special problems. It possibly has to do with "ego-boundaries" and our difficulty in knowing where our own selves end and where our partners' selves begin. My partner should dress in a specific way or should drive in a particular way or should talk more or should talk less … all "shoulds" … all external control. Somewhere in my thinking is the idea that my partner is a reflection on me and should behave accordingly. This control is possibly the biggest threat to the partnership's survival.

Children

If possessiveness becomes a problem in close relationships, parenthood is one role where this happens all too easily. Glasser wrote: "Few of us are prepared to accept that is it our attempts to control that destroys the only thing we have with our children that gives us some control over them, our relationship." He went on to explain the Choice Theory child-rearing axiom as not choosing to do anything that will increase the distance between you and the child, if you want that child to grow up happy and successful.

As loving parents we often unwittingly convert our caring into controlling and the controlling into criticism. It seems to make sense to us to guide our children by letting them know what they are doing wrong (criticism), by gradually shaping them up (controlling) into healthy human beings. The more we try to fix them, the more they need fixing because the relationship is breaking down.

The Destructive Power of Criticism

"I'm only doing it for your own good!" A nurse brandishing a syringe might get away with this remark but it rings false when coming from other sources. We might even have used this phrase once or twice ourselves. It almost always attempts to excuse some form of external control, past, present or threatened. Criticism is one of these "only for your own good" interventions. Perhaps the reason people criticise others is that they do not know of any alternative approach and yet it is one of the major threats to our closest relationships.

Whereas a friend wearing scruffy clothes might be considered funny and we couldn't care less what our enemies wear, we regard a partner or offspring who is untidily dressed as a reflection on our own lives and feel entitled (even compelled) to correct the unacceptable behaviour. Indeed, sometimes it is important that certain behaviours are corrected but criticism is not the best way to do this.

We practise external control in many subtle ways but criticism is its most damaging form. In fact almost any form of judging another human being can be interpreted as an attempt at controlling. "You never leave your room tidy!" "You drive too fast." "You are lazy." "You always come home too late." "You spend too much time with your phone." "You have 20 mistakes in your spelling test."

We do not engage in these criticisms with the friends we meet at the club or in the pub. In fact, Glasser used to joke that the popularity of the pub had a lot to do with the lack of criticism there. It was a criticism-free zone! Where we criticise most is with people who are part of our lives. Whatever the reason for this it is unhealthy for the relationship. We need to know of other ways of dealing with our erring friends, relations and offspring.

Alternatives to Criticism

So what can we do instead? Since we cannot really control another, what can we do when the other's behaviour is somehow unacceptable to us or maybe even dangerous. What can I do if my partner never washes the dishes or my friend drinks too much or my child never looks out for traffic when crossing the road?

The answer lies in respecting the other person's internal control. Ultimately the other person will do what he or she wants to do. All we can do is give them information. However, if they perceive us as being on their side, being friendly and respectful, then they pay more positive attention to what we say. Remember Glasser's advice above about not doing or saying anything that increases the distance between you and the other person.

This means that how we communicate becomes very important. Instead of any form of external control we keep an eye on our relationship, communicate clearly giving information rather than commands. Here are some examples:

- Instead of "You never wash the dishes!" we might say, "We both hate doing the dishes. Let's put on some music and we can do them together."
- Instead of "You come home very late." try, "I love to see you and when you are late I worry about you. I would love you to come home earlier."
- Instead of "Drive more carefully!" we could say, "I know we are different and we drive differently. I like slower speeds and feel more comfortable then."
- Instead of "Stop making noise while I'm trying to work." try, "You two love a good chat. When you do that right beside me I find it hard to concentrate. Would you mind moving to the corner when you want to talk?"
- Instead of "You should have looked both ways before crossing the road" a parent might say, "Tell me what I should do before crossing the road so that I won't be hit by a car or lorry".

- Instead of "You have 20 mistakes in your spelling test" an alternative would be to say, "80% of what you wrote is perfect and English is a difficult language for spelling. Would you like me to show you the correct versions of some of the words?"
- Instead of "You are drinking too much?" a possibility is "If I drink any more it will be bad for me.   Let's head home now" or even "To be honest, I worry about your health when you drink this much."

Common to all these approaches is the idea, "I cannot control you and I don't want to try. I value our relationship and do not want to endanger it." Finding an alternative to criticism does not come easy but this is an ability that improves with practice.

Negotiation

There is a story that teachers of negotiation like to share. It is about a father, an orange and four kids. Dad is not getting peace to read his book in the living room as there are angry voices in the kitchen. He enters to find his four children arguing about an orange each of them wants, and there is only one orange. With the wisdom of Solomon that comes with being a parent he fetches a sharp knife and divides the orange into four very equal pieces to give one to each child, a 25% orange share for each!

All seems well until he passes through the kitchen later and finds a lot of orange pieces scattered across the table.   A family inquisition session follows and strange facts emerge. Niall wanted the rind of the orange to use in a cake. Orla needed the pulp for a biology experiment at school. Susan was keen to see if she could plant the seeds in the garden and poor Patrick only wanted a refreshing glass of orange juice. Dad might be many things but he is not stupid and he quickly realises that each child could have had 100% of what they wanted from the single orange. He had settled for a quick compromise solution of 25% for each.

What could he have done differently? One vital ingredient in conflict resolution is to listen. Understanding each side's needs and wants is a prerequisite for sorting things out together. Another important quality is to believe that solutions better than compromise are often possible but only if we look for them.

Since Choice Theory teaches that we cannot control other people, it encourages us to be respectful of others even where we have a conflict with the other person. Choice Theory recommends the approach, "When we have a problem, we talk about it!" Many schools that follow Glasser's Choice Theory have small posters with this phrase in their classrooms. Notice that it says "WE talk about it" and not "I talk and YOU listen."

Talking is not about arguing, convincing, controlling, criticising. It is about sharing views and looking for a solution that is acceptable to both parties. It is about aiming for the highest possible satisfaction rating for both sides.

- If the problem gives rise to an angry situation it is usually best to wait for this to cool before beginning any negotiation.
- Invite the other person to have a chat about what happened.
- If they are not yet ready for a chat, let them know you will be available later.
- Use the language of collaboration, "Let's talk together." "Let's work something out."
- In a calm way invite the other to explain how they see the problem.
- Listen to them and let them see clearly that you are listening.
- Summarise what you have heard to check that you have understood the other person well.
- Explain how you see the problem.
- Say, "Let's look for a solution that both of us will be happy with."

The Last Resort

Sometimes, no matter how much we wrack our brains, we cannot come up with a positive solution to a relationship problem. The Choice Theory advice for such stalemates is to wait. Work hard to find a solution but if you come to a brick wall, stop banging your head against it. Let some time pass and things might change.

Meanwhile what can you do? There is actually something quite positive you can do and it is based on taking a different view of the problem. Do you know how to make this relationship problem worse? Think about it. There are probably quite a number of ways you could really stir up trouble. Next question: Do you want to make it worse? My guess is that you do not.

So here is the choice you have, the choice not to make things any worse. What will that look like? What situations are likely to arise where it would be easy to make things worse? How are you going to deal with them? Imagining them in advance and planning your strategy for dealing with them is the best way to keep the relationship from suffering more. Although this plan sounds somewhat negative at first, what you are choosing to do is in fact to behave in a peaceful way, to protect the relationship.

A World of Better Relationships

The more people understand Choice Theory and use it in their lives, the less we will see attempts by one person to control another. In any relationship, a partnership, a family, a school, where Choice Theory is explicitly adopted as a guide to behaviour, the relationships will not be free of all problems but the solving process will be smoother.

Glasser wrote that, "external control is more widely used in marriage than in any other relationship. In contrast, external control is almost never used in a long-term friendship. In fact, long-term friendships are the only human relationships where, without knowing that we are doing it, we use choice theory from the start."

The firm conviction that we cannot control another person and that to do so damages the relationship is the key to getting on well together.

8. Managing Your Time

Someone once described Ireland as the land of "time enough". Our relaxed attitude to time can be endearing but taking life at a wise pace should not be confused with taking life at no pace at all. Time is not simply something that happens in a clock or watch. Time is life and your time is your life. Time is also one of the ways we link our lives to other people. Mismanage time and you are messing up your life, a sure formula for stress.

It is a characteristic of the so-called "Type-A Personality" never to have enough time, to be trying to do more than one thing at once, to be stressed and to have an increased risk of heart failure. In spite of the obvious importance of reasonable skill at time-management, we are not often taught about it nor attempt to learn it for ourselves.

As a teenager at school in Belfast I took time very seriously. So seriously in fact that I would spend a lot of my study time drafting complex study timetables. The problem was that, by the time the schedule was drawn up, there was no time left for study. The fact of the matter is that time-management does not begin with time nor even with a diary or timetable. It begins with deciding what you want, what you really want. Having an advanced agenda system with no clear idea of what you want is like having a wonderful fast car but no map!

Clarify What You Really Want

When you complain about not having enough time, what you really mean is that you do not have enough time to do what you really want to do. So it makes good logical sense to start your new approach to time-management by looking at what you really want to do with your time. These are the quality world pictures of Choice Theory psychology, the important ways you have chosen to meet your basic needs.

If we do not take the trouble to identify our important wants, real life places a range of minor tasks in our path and these can easily use up valuable time. Some of these tasks may be important but, unless we allocate time for what are priority items for us, we may not leave sufficient time for them.

One of the longest words in the English language is "Yes". When someone asks you to do something for them and you say "yes", you are in fact allocating time from your life to that particular task. It makes sense to agree to doing things that you really want to do. However, it is not always easy to say "no" to a friend or colleague.

Dr. Glasser had his own recommendation for such awkward occasions. He suggested we would reply saying, "I need time to think about that!" This is neither a "yes" or a "no" but shares with the other person that you give importance to their request and, at the same time, that you have some difficulty with it. I recall saying this to a colleague who was inviting me to give a presentation. When he saw I needed to think about it, he quickly explained that he was asking me first out of courtesy but he had another person lined up too. I heaved a sigh of relief ... and maybe he did too!

We need to bring some focus on what you want. We are not referring to your overall plan for the rest of your life. What are the really important things you want to do in the next week? Jotting these down on a piece of paper is a good way to improve the focus. Even better, enter the events straight into your time-management control system!

Stephen Covey, one of the great experts on time-management, relates a demonstration he witnessed involving rocks, pebbles, sand and water. If you put the rocks in the container first you can still fit in the pebbles, sand and even water. Start with the sand or pebbles and there will be no room for the rocks. In time management terms it means we need to timetable our big rocks first, the things we really want.

Covey recommended doing this type of prioritising once a week. A good first step towards better time-management would be to choose a time right now for this weekly review session. It might be first thing on a Monday morning or around mid-day on a Saturday, for example.

Allocate a Time for This

The next step is to choose a time to do each of these important items, your personal big rocks, and to enter this plan straight into your diary or whichever method you use to remind yourself later on. There is no ideal approach for this as it depends on what suits your preferences and your life-style. Very few people can rely simply on their memory! Here are some of the options:

- Sticky Notes: These are quite flexible but are limited to a specific location such as your desk.
- Cards: Small index cards can be both flexible and portable but date and time might not be so easy to manage. These can be especially useful for managing a local task such as homework or study.
- Paper Calendar: Date and time are easier to identify on a calendar but it is tied to a specific location. This can be useful where event details need to be shared with a group.
- Diary: A book diary is portable and reasonably flexible, probably the system that suits the majority of people who wish to manage their time better.
- Computer Calendar: Data entry needs a little more care than with paper equivalents but such calendars usually have alarms and can sometimes be synchronised across several devices, even those belonging to different members of a team or family.

Carry out Your Plan

Do what you decided to do. At some point in our lives we come to the amazing realisation that writing something down is not the same as doing it. If I decide to write an important letter at 8 pm on Tuesday, then that is what I should be doing at 8 pm on Tuesday. If, in the light of more recent plans, I realise I cannot do this at that time, then I can easily reschedule it. This fine-tuning requires its own planning.

Have a time for planning the day. Some people prefer to do this on the previous afternoon or evening. Others prefer to take the first ten minutes or so of the new day. The time allocations you set in your diary a few days ago may require minor adjustments. You find you have free time at 10 am and decide to do the 8 pm letter in that morning slot. Rigidly adhering to your earlier plan would be foolish but the fact of having a plan means you can adjust it more effectively and stay in control of your time.

Depending on your personal life-style, it can be very helpful to segment your day on a regular basis. For example, have a time for revising your plan, a time for reading your mail, a segment for making calls to other premises. Those who engage in writing usually find a particular time of day better for their more creative work and other times better for proof-reading.

Mark Completed Tasks

It is good for your self-esteem to put a tick at tasks you have completed. This is easy on paper calendars or diaries and some electronic diaries have this facility. It is generally not a good idea to erase completed items since a historical record of what you have done can be useful for lots of reasons.

Take Adequate Breaks

There is a certain logic about thinking, "I don't have time to have a break" but the logic is wrongl A snack break mid-morning and mid-afternoon together with a reasonable lunch break are not only important for physical nourishment. They also help the mind refreshen and overall productivity improves. Recalling a cartoon I saw recently, write the word "nothing" here and there in your "to-do" list and remember to put a tick at it when you do it!

Drive Slowly

The famous racing driver James Hunt was once asked how did he manage to drive so fast. He replied that he in fact drove very slowly, acknowledging that it was the car that went fast. When we have planned something well, we enact our plan on schedule and we pace ourselves well, we do not "hurry" in our mind's eye. Ignore good planning and we tend to hurry through life scurrying from one panic to the next.

Reduce Clutter

One of the big unwelcome consumers of our time is clutter and one of the biggest contributors to this is email.

- Do not subscribe to any notifications without due thought.
- Unsubscribe from emails you do not want (unless they are spam).
- Use an email provider that filters out most spam.
- Report any spam that does reach you.
- Get into the habit of deleting unimportant emails swiftly.
- If an email is important, put the action required straight into your diary.
- Have a set time, ideally at the start of the day, when you check work-related emails, sorting them as you read through them.

Control Phone Calls

Another form of clutter is the telephone and the modern version of this follows us wherever we go. It's a great little stress machine to carry through life!

- Do not give people your telephone number readily.
- Remember: you do not have to answer any phone ever!
- Never give a phone priority over a real live person.

- Don't answer it when it's not convenient for you.
- Take it off the hook or switch to "silent".
- Don't use an answering machine or, if you do, never say "I'll phone you back".
- Always use call identifying and ignore non-identifiable calls.
- When arranging a call with someone tell them when to phone you.
- Assign all your pre-arranged calls to a narrow slot of time.
- Make it clear to people that you do not like telephone calls at certain times, e.g., after 9pm or on week-ends.
- Associate a special ring tone to numbers that can be "awkward".
- Only use "Call Interrupt" if you like having many calls and interruptions!
- Know how to end phone conversations (e.g. using a summary).

From a Choice Theory perspective, your time is yours. As is true about life in general, you have more choices than you might realise. Setting aside different times to plan your choices means setting time for you to run your own life. Poor time management can lead to pile-ups of things to do, a sure recipe for stress.

Control Chat

It can be very nice to have a short chat with friends from time to time but most of us have experience of people who just chat on and on and on. Whether this is on the telephone, over the garden fence or at the water fountain at work, it can seriously reduce the time we have available for other matters. There is an art in ending a conversation and here are some guidelines.

- Give a closure signal such as, "It was lovely meeting you!"
- Simply say, "I need to go now".
- Refer to the next time you will talk.
- Give a short summary of any points raised or actions planned.

So, to summarise, I have explained the importance of attending first to our priorities, of having planning times, of care with clutter and phones and of knowing how to end a conversation. Will catch up with you again in the next chapter!

9. Getting enough Sleep

Airport security screens are not intended for public viewing but it is hard not to notice them on our way through. An amazing change in recent years is the amount of cables that people are carrying in their hand luggage. My guess is that most of these are charging cables for the array of portable devices that have become part of our basic needs and, indeed, part of our new nightly before-bed ritual.

The more important daily charging does not require any cables at all and here I am referring to sleep, the body's way of restoring lost energy in readiness for a new day. For many people it is easy enough to fall asleep during the day and equally easy to fall awake at night! Life is not fair.

If you really want to become stressed even by minor frustrations then one of the best ways to do this is to neglect your sleep. Attempting to manage your life with debilitated physical and mental powers greatly increases the possibility of stress. All your special talents and acquired abilities take a hammering if you have not fuelled up your life with adequate rest.

To make matters worse, once we do get stressed we find it harder to sleep and easier to wake up during the night. So what choices do we have with regard to our sleep?

Give Sleep a Chance

Having a set bed-time is important since your body's expectation to sleep at a certain time facilitates the whole process of sleeping. Avoid napping during the day. Make sure you get some good physical exercise during the day as that makes night sleep easier. Avoid eating and drinking just before your bedtime, ideally in the previous three hours, and avoid alcohol, caffeine and nicotine especially in the evening.

Do what you can to create a restful atmosphere in your bedroom and do not use it for work of any kind. If you are a student and the only place you can study is your bedroom, try to separate bed and desk as much as possible but never, ever study (or do any work) in bed.

As bedtime approaches, avoid using your mobile phone or computers as the bluish screen light is not conducive to sleep. In particular avoid exciting games and news updates. On the other hand many people find a little light reading in bed conducive to sleep since it can help create a buffer between day's work and the night's rest.

Do not Try to Sleep

Counting sheep and other popular techniques for falling asleep all suffer from one major contradiction. They involve trying and deliberate effort of any kind is diametrically opposed to any form of relaxation. It's like fighting for peace!

Tossing and turning do not help either as these brusque movements arouse the body even more. So, get into a comfortable position and then take slow deep breaths.

If your mind is occupied by thoughts of problems, do not attempt to banish them from your head. Instead, do your best to replace them with thoughts of something pleasant. You can choose what to think about. Ask yourself if thinking about your problems in bed will do any good.

For more persistent problem an idea is to jot down a summary in a notebook kept by your bed for that very purpose with the idea of attending to them during the day. Do not worry about not falling asleep. Remind yourself that, provided you stay lying down without tossing and turning, you are resting.

Waking up at Night

One of the problems with waking during the night is that many people assume they are supposed to be asleep all night! Although we may have the impression that our nights are normally one long deep sleep, in fact that is not the case. We drift in and out of deep sleep during the night. This happens about every 90 minutes or so for most people. Sometimes, in the lighter periods, we waken up. This in itself is not a problem.

Instead of worrying about the lack of sleep, remind yourself that you are in fact resting and that waking up a few times during the night is not necessarily bad. You might not have had much choice about waking up during the night but you can choose how to view this and you can choose what you are going to do about it.

Effects of Drugs

Almost any drugs, including the prescribed variety, can disturb normal sleep patterns. Instead of the multiple phases of sleep mentioned above, drugs can induce one much deeper slumber that is not so good for our rest, not to mention the other effects (sometimes oddly called "side-effects") they may engender.

Treat Sleep as Important

Sleep is our personal recharging time and, as such, it is very important. Not getting enough rest or even keeping irregular hours can all lead to a less restful sleep and ultimately we pay the price in reduced energy and alertness. It is so easy to "burn the candle at both ends" just before examinations or the conclusion of an important project. Better study skills and planning right from the beginning of an academic year can help offset this last minute abandonment of adequate sleep.

10. Work

I want to know your name and I want to know what you do! We all tend to seek these two facts on meeting a person for the first time. Somehow or other we assume that knowing a person's job tells us a lot about him or her. Of course, a person's identity involves a lot of other things: values, feelings, thoughts, plans and hopes, hobbies and interests, beliefs and fears, and even physical appearance.

Still, knowing what a person "does" seems to help us get to know them better. My occupation even becomes part of my own identity. After all, it is how we spend a significant part of our lives and it tends to create a special network of acquaintances we meet daily.

If my working life is not in good shape, then a sizeable part of my whole life is unsatisfactory. Since Choice Theory psychology sees stress as the signal telling us that something is not working well for us, it makes sense to examine some of the areas in our work where our needs are not satisfied. There is no shortage of these!

Getting There

Many workers are already exhausted by the time they arrive at their place of employment. A long journey or driving through heavy traffic is energy sapping. It is worthwhile giving specific time to a search for alternatives: a different route, another mode of transport, car sharing. If using public transport, it can prove more relaxing if the trip is spent listening to music or reading a novel. You have a choice to see your journey as a horrible chore, a waste of time, a traffic nightmare or to see it as an opportunity to do things you like.

Sometimes, choosing a different departure time (earlier or later) can result in a shorter or more pleasant journey. In fact, leaving home even a few minutes earlier might make the difference between a relaxed start to the day and a nail-biting start. Aiming to be early rather than punctual can do a lot for peace of mind. In extreme situations it may be worth considering a change of dwelling or even a change of job if the journey to work seems unavoidably tiresome.

Influencing your Boss

If you have been reading the earlier portions of this book you will know by now that you cannot control your boss! So what are your options? What can you do when you are keen to do a good job well but your boss's ideas, methods or whatever keep getting in the way? A boss can make life difficult for you by being too bossy, too fussy, overly critical, abusive, chatty (as in time-wasting), remote.

Years ago I was talking to Dr. Glasser after he had addressed a big gathering of conference attendees and members of the public in Galway. A lady approached and asked him if he had any ideas for dealing with school principals. Now this was a topic that I was interested in too so I took note of his answer. Almost without delay he replied, "Don't go to your principal with problems; go with solutions".

For example, instead of reporting constant photo-copy breakdowns to your superior, you might suggest that the machine would be more reliable if placed under the supervision of a member of staff who is nearby. You and others at the front-line tend to know more about possible solutions than any manager. Becoming part of the solution rather than the bearer of bad news will be appreciated by your superior and contributes to team spirit.

Where a superior's own personality or habits are causing problems for you, you may need a more complex approach. A first phase would be to establish good relations with your boss insofar as this is possible. The next phase requires diplomacy and skill. Assertiveness is the art of respecting the other's needs while respecting your own at the same time. You could say to your boss: "When you keep telling me what to do I really appreciate your experience but I feel nervous, as if you do not trust me completely". Notice that this is not a criticism; it simply explains that when YOU do X, I feel Y. It is giving your superior some information.

Too Much Work

It is remarkably easy to get totally caught up in work, going non-stop from early morning to late evening. As stress levels increase, the ability to think clearly diminishes and with it the hope of a solution fades.

Any advice that includes "work less" is unlikely to be helpful or heeded. What is vital is to take rest-breaks. Paradoxically these can increase your productivity rather than diminish it. The break does have to be a real change and not simply work with a cup of coffee instead of work without a cup of coffee. You may need some convincing about this, so start with a five-minute break, one where you leave your work location and do something totally different. A quick walk outside the building or a friendly chat with a co-worker are examples. Whatever you do it should be a positive activity. According to Choice Theory psychology, changing your doing or thinking will also mean a change in your feeling and physiology and you will return to work with a fresher total behaviour.

Another break that is vital here is what we might call a "reflective break", one where you allow time to reflect on what you have been doing. Work out what tasks you need to do and what interruptions impede you. Writing this down can be important. For each of the things that mess up your work, consider what you could do to change this. If you cannot come up with solutions it can help to consult with someone else. When speeding along under the influence of stress, the thinking component of our behaviour tends to be neglected so slow down and give it some space.

Before applying for a promotion it makes sense to check if you are ready for the extra challenges. Advice I gleaned from the internet is "Never buy a car you can't push". By all means go for promotion but prepare for the extra responsibilities.

Interruptions

It always seems that when you have most to do, you get most interruptions: people, phones, email! It would be easy, so easy to be rude to people who interrupt you a lot but good relationships are important in the workplace. Instead of a straight rejection, offer a later appointment: "Can you call back at 12:30?"

A good gatekeeper such as a well-trained secretary can do a lot to offset unnecessary telephone calls. A call identifier system can help you judge whether an incoming call is important or not. As a last resort offering a later time slot can help here too. Whether you answer the phone or not is always your choice.

Emails are a marvellous invention but many of us suffer from an excess of these. A good filtering and labelling system in your email program can help you focus on the more important emails. An early morning session of ruthless deletion of non-relevant emails can become a daily digital desktop clearing that helps you attend to the important messages.

Some "interruptions" are hard to ignore as when a colleague asks you to do something for them. It is very difficult to say "no" even when you know you need to. Glasser recommended saying, "I need to think about that" in these situations. This communicates your interest in helping but also your difficulty in doing so.

Understanding Others

We all know people who are constantly greedy for power, hungry for affection, people who value their freedom dearly or those who always seem to be on the look out for fun. Glasser defines these general inclinations in people as "needs intensities" and they can help us understand work colleagues and even superiors.

My way of picturing the normal functioning of the basic needs is to imagine them as batteries that should be kept well charged. If my fun need is running low (due to sitting through a long boring lecture), my behavioural system gets frustration signals (equivalent to a "low charge" warning light) urging it to come up with some fun-need satisfying behaviour (a recharge). As a result I might choose to daydream for a while or to send a funny text message to a friend. I succeed in recharging my fun battery and all is well again in that department.

The concept of needs intensities fits the battery model very well. Imagine each individual having five batteries (corresponding to the five needs) but not all are the same size. For one person the power battery is much bigger than the rest and so this individual is characterised by a constant search for power. This may result in a constant hunger for knowledge, a quest for leadership, a strongly competitive spirit or even in an attempt to achieve power over people.

Where this concept of needs intensities becomes interesting is when we analyse a group of people who spend a lot of time together. By way of example, pick your immediate superior, yourself and perhaps two other work colleagues. Guess at the needs intensities of each rating them from one to ten on each of the needs where ten indicates a very strong need.

Almost immediately you will see how each has an agenda that stems from his or her needs intensities profile. Here is an example: Mary has a high power need intensity and so has Michael. They constantly come into conflict often over trivial matters such as who sits where in the canteen. Their boss is Karen whose main need intensity is for love and belonging. Her efforts to be kind to Mary achieve little in the way of recognition. Ben has a strong constant need for freedom and, since Karen's kindness results in him getting plenty of space to work at his own pace, he is a happy worker.

Square Pegs in Square Holes

One of my own immediate bosses had a knack of team leadership second to none. Essentially what he did was to put square pegs in square holes. He would focus on the strengths of an individual and then seek a place in the team where these strengths could flourish. This contrasts sharply with attempts to squeeze square pegs into round holes, with criticism and even punishment of the pegs for not fitting!

From a Choice Theory perspective, this boss was ensuring maximum need satisfaction for each worker. This created a happy workplace and one that was amazingly productive in every way. One measure of the shape of each "peg" could be the person's needs intensities profile. Other important dimensions would be the person's special abilities and interests (quality world).

For a work environment to be truly need-satisfying, the management team needs to be committed to achieving this, they need to listen, to get to know the team very well. For a start, the manager needs to know the shape of the pegs and the shape of the holes.

In fact, there are two characteristics of the need-satisfying workplace: the relationships and the work itself. We work better with people we like and we work better with work we like.

The Boss and the Leader

Although I have been referring to the "boss" above, Glasser distinguished carefully between a boss and a leader. The "boss" believes in external control and so his or her whole approach is centred on control. The boss tells people what to do and how to do it, uses rewards or even threats and constantly evaluates the work done. A "leader", on the other hand, discusses the work and procedures with the employees, works with them rather than over them and invites them to evaluate their own work. Leadership fosters team spirit and job satisfaction.

From an employer's point of view, choosing a "boss" approach generates a lot of stress since people resist being controlled. The constant supervision, trust issues, and disputes about demarcation all contribute to an atmosphere of tension and even fear. Where there is a "boss", there is stress for everyone, including the "boss".

Retirement

Some people spend a lot of their working lives dreaming of the "carefree" days of retirement with lots of time for the beach, the golf-course or the pub. In some respects it might be carefree but it is not without its own variety of stress.

Consider for a moment how need-fulfilling work can be. The responsibilities of work and the satisfaction of a job well done can do a lot for our power needs. Relationships with fellow-workers and even with our clients help meet our belonging need. Fun is to be found in the excitement of new products, projects or services. The financial rewards for work contribute greatly to what we do in our free time and to our general survival need. All of these satisfactions can disappear immediately after retirement and for some that shock can be quite traumatic.

The knowledge and skills you fought so hard to obtain together with the reputation that you acquired as a result, all these now tend to gather dust on a shelf. You begin to see yourself as different from the person that was, the person that went to work every day, who was called upon to deal with challenging situations. The more job specific your skills the more likely you are to feel the void that is left.

On facing into retirement it becomes vital to plan new ways of meeting or managing your needs and of using your skills or a new version of them. Doing charity work, joining clubs, new interests, consultancy work, travel - all can help. There is no unique formula that suits everybody except that everyone needs to make their own choices about these issues when they retire.

Unemployment

Any time spent without a job can have a similar negative effect on your basic needs and a corresponding risk of feeling stressed. Apart from the sense of a gap in your own identity, a series of failed attempts to find work can gradually grind us down. We can depress and stress at that same time; depressing about the apparent hopelessness of unemployment and stressing about the difficulties in surviving.

There is no simple effective solution to this but there is one simple solution that can be guaranteed not to work: do nothing!

It can help to have more realistic expectations, knowing that making a few job applications are unlikely to be enough, that it may take dozens of attempts. Similarly it can be beneficial to anticipate that many applications will be refused or, worse still, ignored and it is unpleasant to feel rejected. One healthy way to counter this constant stream of negative feedback is to engage in voluntary work. Helping counter the constant "no job" messages will be expressions of gratitude, feelings of satisfaction and comradeship. There are the added advantages of gaining work experience and showing a willingness to work, two characteristics that enhance employment prospects.

All Work and No Play

Yes indeed, all work and no play makes Jack a dull boy and Jill a dull girl! Worse still, it can make them both very stressed. As I have mentioned above, rest periods have a very important role in a working day. There are other activities that are equally important. Social meetings with work colleagues and superiors have a vital role in creating a happy work place. The occasional staff party, competition, sports outing or birthday celebrations all help to humanise the work place. Even in-service training tends to have beneficial effects far beyond the training content.

Informal friendly contact fosters an atmosphere where problems that arise can be treated in a collaborative spirit and where creative ideas can be proposed without fear of ridicule or criticism.

People can also work together to enhance their work environment. Careful colour and lighting schemes, pictures, flower, background music all can help if appropriate.

The basic Choice Theory attitude to any situation is to look at the choices we have. Work related stress, like any form of stress, might be helped temporarily by some breathing exercises but is more likely to benefit from addressing the actual causes of the stress. When it is not clear what the causes are, an analysis of the basic needs can be useful. Choice Theory does not attempt to offer specific solutions and those I offer above are only provided as examples. What Choice Theory psychology does emphasise is that stress is a feeling and as such is warning us that we are not meeting our needs. Consequently we need to do something about it and the first step is to identify the problems and find out how to solve them.

11. Checking Your Basic Needs

Eileen's problem was that Eileen did not know what Eileen's problem was. There was nothing obvious. She had a good job with a decent salary, a nice house and good friends. Of late she seemed to take longer getting to sleep, lying there for ages with eyes wide open, her mind stuck in a psychological waste-land somewhere between stress and despair. It would have been easy for her to believe that she had been "infected" by a mental illness or the dreaded "ennui" of the philosophers she had read in her university days.

A chance remark by a work colleague about "getting her basic needs checked out" inspired Eileen to scribble a few ideas in her diary during the morning coffee break. "Survival: all well. Power: doing well at work. Freedom: can do what I want. Love and Belonging: very good friends. Fun: ????" That fun need stumped Eileen. Yes, she had smiled her way through a few sit-coms on the television in recent times but she could not remember when she last had a really good laugh.

The more she thought about it the more she realised that her life had been just too comfortable with nothing new or exciting in recent times. Time to talk to Maria, she thought, Maria being the zaniest of her friends. That resulted in a meeting in a new oriental restaurant down the street, plans for a week-end together in Paris and an application for promotion at work. Life began to sparkle again.

In this book we have attempted to identify some of the typical causes of stress in adults but sometimes the causes of our stress are not so obvious and some personal psychological probing is required. The basic needs described in Choice Theory provide a useful framework for such a self-examination. These offer a quick guide to the main pillars of your personal well-being and a handy structure for analysing your life-style.

Choice Theory psychology teaches that in almost all we do we are striving to meet our basic needs. By "needs" we mean whatever it is that you must have, something that is essential for your life. For example, we all need food but we do not specifically need potatoes. We could survive by eating something else other than potatoes provided we meet the need for food (survival).

In our daily lives we do not go around thinking specifically about our needs. Instead we focus on the ways we might meet the needs, ways that Glasser called pictures in our Quality Worlds. So, when we feel hungry (the need for survival), we look around for some sort of food that we like. Similarly we plan to meet friends, save for a new car, watch a comedy on the television and a host of other daily activities. What we are always doing, mainly subconsciously, is striving to meet our basic needs.

We can in fact use these needs in a more conscious way to examine our lives, to see how well we are doing. This can be especially important if we are stressed but are not sure why.

Read through the following outline of the basic needs and use the questions to estimate how well you are satisfying each need. Pay particular attention to areas that are not going well for you since these are most likely contributing to your stress. The questions are not intended to be exhaustive but offer a sample of the areas included in each need.

Love and Belonging

This is the need for human warmth, contact, intimacy or simply connectedness to other human beings.

- How many good friends do you have right now?
- Are your relationships going well, especially the most important ones?
- Do you spend real time with friends at least a few times a week?
- Are you involved in any clubs, community activities and the like?

Power

This is like the power of a battery, a sense of inner strength that comes from your personal control of your life.

- Do you feel in reasonable control of your life now, at home, at work, at school?
- Do people really listen to you?
- Are your skills and knowledge recognised by others?
- Are you aware of your own worth as a person?
- Do you feel competent enough for the job you are doing (or examinations you will do)?

Freedom

This is the need to be able to move and do things as you wish, not to feel fettered or limited in what you try to do.

- Are you able to run your life as you wish?
- Do you feel that others attempt to control you?
- Are there restraints on your life now due to money or other circumstances?
- Do you have adequate breaks for work or study during the day?
- Do you have regular holidays or days off?
- Do you have some time everyday that you can really call your own?

Fun

This is more than a simple decoration of life, some sort of luxury. It is the sparkle that accompanies new experiences and new learning or new views of our situation. Glasser associated it very strongly with learning which is how we cope with and adapt to our ever-changing world.

- Do you have something to laugh about each day?
- Do you have fun with some of your regular contacts?
- Is there something exciting or new going on in your life?
- Do you have something to look forward to right now?
- Do you have hopes or plans for the immediate future?

Survival

This need includes personal health and safety, comfort, food and nourishment.

- Do you have sufficient food?
- Are you getting enough healthy food and drink?
- Do you engage in some form of exercise (e.g., walking) almost every day?
- Do you have a reasonably comfortable home?
- Do you have sufficient money to live as you wish?
- Are you fairly healthy?
- Do you feel safe?

Make a quick summary

Now that you have some understanding of the basic needs, give yourself a score on each, a percentage that reflects how well you are meeting each of the needs.

- Love & Belonging
- Power
- Freedom
- Fun
- Survival

If one or more needs has a low score, it is time to consider what specifically you could be doing to satisfy these needs better. Tim was surprised to find that he had marked his power need as low. He recently had a promotion, one that gave him responsibility for leading a team and he now realised that he felt very far from content in his new role. The confidence he had at work before his promotion had now petered away.

He could decide that he was not cut out for his new leadership role but he made a different choice. He thought, "I don't know enough about leading so I had better learn something about it". The negative feeling helped him see a gap in his knowledge and skills and so he decided to fill that gap.

What can you do?

An assessment of your needs can give you a general idea of where your stresses originate. You still need to probe more and find the specific frustrations. If, for example, you sense that your freedom need is not being met well, it may be that you have totally neglected this area of your life or that your attempts to meet the need have been unsuccessful. You join a club to get a rest from work but end up entangled in club administration! If what you are choosing to do is not meeting your needs then it is time to change it.

This is not always an easy process and sometimes it is good to consult with someone else. Whatever it is, only you can take the next step.

From Needs to Action

The frustration that is at the root of stress is ultimately a signal for action. Just as physical pain urges a diagnosis and a remedy so too does the psychological pain of frustration. We manage our stress by heeding the signal and choosing what to do about it. We ask ourselves questions such as these:

Which of my needs seems to be running low at present? (e.g., love and belonging)

What specifically is lacking or missing? (e.g., not taking time for recreation with my family)

What have I been doing so far to meet this need and how well is it working?

What relatively simple action could I choose to do soon that would meet my need? (e.g., arrange a family visit to a favourite restaurant in the next few days.)

Thinking of your needs as if they were your private set of batteries used to run your life can be a helpful image. You ask yourself, "what can I choose to charge up my batteries right now?"

Sometimes it can be difficult to make a decision, a choice or to plan the implementation of that choice. We address these issues in the next chapter.

12. Decisions and Plans

There is an old joke about the chap who said, "I used to be indecisive but now I'm unsure". We have all been at that place in our lives but how in fact do you know what makes a good decision? Obviously a good outcome is a reliable measure of the quality of a decision but the question I really want to ask is, "how do you know what makes a good decision beforehand?" How can you ensure that the decision you are about to make has the highest probability of a good outcome?

After all, if you have identified the causes of your stress your next step will be to make decisions and plans to take charge of your life again. A poorly constructed decision or plan will be less effective in reducing your stress and might even increase it.

Good Decisions

So what are some of the key ingredients in making the best possible decision about choices for the future?

WANTS: Be clear about what you want to achieve with your decision. That means being as specific as you can. For example, it might be about a short holiday. Is the decision about choosing a holiday that is good for you or for you plus your partner or for you plus your family? What does a "good holiday" look like? What are the key characteristics you are looking for? For one person the cost might be a vital factor, for another the proximity of a beach.

OPTIONS: Consider as many options as you can. This may mean asking around, doing a little research, using the internet. At first glance there may be only two ways of dealing with a difficult neighbour: fight or flight. After some research you realise that negotiation is yet another option.

INFORMATION: Get as much information as you can about each option on your short list. Look for hard evidence such as the experience of others. Take into account any bias that your information source might have. A holiday brochure might show you the best view of the hotel taken when freshly painted and on a sunny day and avoiding the noisy railway line alongside!

PROS AND CONS: List the pros (potential benefits) and cons (potential negative consequences) of each of the options. The better your research, the more complete will be your list of pros and cons. It's a good idea to write down the options together with the pros and cons and revisit your list over a period of time. The more important the decision, the more advisable it is to write down your analysis of it.

PRIORITISE: Underline or encircle the pros and cons that are most important for you.

REVERSABILITY: Take into consideration whether any given option is reversible or not. In other words, if you choose that option and find that it's not working out well, can you change to another option? For example, choosing to emigrate to the far side of the world would be hard to reverse.

CONSULT: If possible share your list with a good friend who may be able to add options, pros or cons. If the decision will involve another person (e.g., a partner), share as much as possible with that person before arriving at your final decision.

CHOOSE: You could spend the rest of your life on any decision but normally you will have a date or time when you need to make a choice. The more research you have put into the preparation for your decision the easier it will be to make the choice with confidence. If you still find it hard to choose, then you need more information about your options.

Good Plans

Once you have decided on a course of action the next step is to plan that well. Knowing what to do is not enough. It is vital to know how to do it also. Here are some of the characteristics of good plans:

PREPARATION: Planning means working in advance and this in itself requires time. Make this clear to yourself by sitting down with pencil and paper. Listing the things you need to do will help you decide on a time-line for them.

PRIORITIES: What are the bigger issues that usually need to be addressed first? Spend some time determining the sequence of events. Preparation for a job interview, for example, may require a few days library research, shopping for some new clothes, a visit to the hairdresser, leave home at 8 am to be at least 30 minutes early for your 11 am interview. It is a good idea to allow some extra time for the unexpected.

POSSIBLE: Choose something you really can do and will do. Aim for at least 90% success. Absolutely anyone can tear a telephone directory in two … if they tear out one page at a time! If you think your plan might not work, adjust it so that you become fairly certain it will work.

PRECISE: Make the plan as specific as possible. Check out all the details: what? Where? When? Who with? How? For example: "What is the best time to talk to your friend about this?", "Where will you meet?", "How will you open the conversation; what exact words will you use?"

POSITIVE: Decide what you are going to do rather than what you are not going to do. Aim to start something rather than stop something. Instead of "I will stop wasting time" you might say "I will start my work at eight o'clock".

PROMPT: Do it now … or even sooner! Starting as soon as possible has several advantages. It allows you time to adjust if necessary. It also means you have time to spare if some of your plans get delayed.

PRACTICE: Once you have decided on an action, rehearse what you are going to do. In preparing for a job interview, for example, practise walking into a room and sitting down comfortably. Practise saying your opening words and drill yourself in a few variations of these. All of this builds confidence and also helps you spot problems in advance.

PROMISE: Make a strong commitment to yourself. If you are saying "I'll try" or "I might" adjust your plan so that you can say "I will". "I'll try to study for 4 hours each day" becomes, "I will study for 1 hour each day".

PROTECT: Protect your plan. Anticipate potential sabotage. Check that there is not something else important at the time you intend carrying out your plan. A good plan for an important appointment at 9 am might be scuppered if you forget that the school on route to your appointment has parental traffic jams every day at that time.

PROCESS: Evaluate the effectiveness of your plan as you put it into operation and after you have completed it. Simply ask yourself, "How well did my plan work?", "Do I need to adjust anything?"

PERSEVERANCE: Keep trying. In the follow-up do not spend time on excusing, blaming, moaning or criticising. The only real failure is to give up trying. Think in terms of what you need to change to make your plan work.

Why not try this now? Make a simple plan for something you will do today. Then check each of the qualities above to see how well your plan matches up. Do not use these ideas for marriage proposals just yet; learn your skill with simple plans at first.

13. Emergency Strategies

Someone once defined stress as to wake up screaming and then realise you hadn't fallen asleep yet! Stress can knock us for six! It can feel like a wave of electrical currents racing through our bodies, currents that are frightening and make it virtually impossible to rest or sleep.

With this full tsunami effect of stress we are in a state of shock and probably in no shape just yet to analyse the situation or think about solutions. For these critical moments we need to have a range of emergency strategies, things we can do to help deal with the initial sensation of overwhelm.

Many authors offer such strategies as "ways to deal with stress" but I believe they are more accurately described as "ways to get ready to deal with stress". Be aware that none of these options will in themselves address the causes of our stress. They simply help us regain our strength so that we become more able to tackle the origins of our stress.

These are all examples of the "Choice Time" introduced earlier. You may not know what to do in the longer term but you can choose to do something now, an activity that will give you the added energy you need to deal more directly with the frustrations.

Safeguard Your Health

If you have or suspect you have any health issues that could be worsened by stress, consult with a doctor about what to do. A sudden surge of stress is not good for anyone with delicate physical health and a medical intervention could be important.

Get Some Rest

In severe stress it may be difficult to fall off to sleep. However, rest is still a possibility. The trouble is that whatever is causing the stress can easily invade the mind at such times. Rest is not limited to the sit or lie down variety. Choosing to do something totally different for a short time may be as good as a rest.

Listen to Music

Everyone has their own taste in this. For some, the more relaxing the music the better but others prefer music that will almost overpower their senses, music for submersion!

Do Breathing Exercises

Many authors recommend deep breathing exercises for stressful moments. This can certainly be helpful but it is important that this be slow. When experiencing stress you may be breathing more rapidly than normal so it is helpful to slow it down gradually. Any fast movements, including fast breathing, are likely to increase the adrenalin rush in your body.

Use Water Therapy

Water comes in many forms and almost all of them are soothing to the person with stress. Cold water splashed about the face, a shower, a bath, a walk in the rain, a stroll along the beach, paddling at the water's edge, a sauna or jacuzzi. Swimming is not only good water therapy but is also an excellent all-round exercise.

Do Some Exercise

Almost any fully engrossing activity can be equivalent of a full body massage and this can help shake up tense muscles throughout the body. Football, swimming, tennis, sailing and a host of other sports offer activities that can also give the mind a rest from the worries that are generating the stress. For some people more gentle forms of exercise are better: yoga, tai chi, pilates. For almost everyone a short walk in the fresh air is good for body and mind. If it's cold, wear a coat; if it's raining use a raincoat.

Charge Your Energy

It is very easy to neglect basics such as food and general self-care when stress appears to have taken over. Even if you do not know what to do about the stress itself, it makes sense to build up your body by eating adequately and drinking plenty of water. That could become the motto of this chapter: when you do not know what to do that will help, do something positive anyway!

Have a Laugh

Under the dark cloud of stress it can be hard to watch a gripping drama on the screen. What is more likely to hold our attention is a good comedy. The ability to laugh at these times can be quite a tonic. Pick some comedy that has a tried and tested record for you and view it again preferably in the company of a partner or friends.

Learn to Relax

Relaxing is not something most people can do at will. We can easily lift our arms and wriggle our toes but relaxing does not seem to be something we can order ourselves to do. The reason is simple. "Trying" to do anything is quite the opposite of relaxing. Trying to relax, similar to trying to sleep, is likely to achieve quite the opposite effect.

It was precisely this paradoxical effect that led Dr. Edmund Jacobson to develop his "progressive relaxation" technique in the 1920's. The full details are readily available at different locations on the internet but you can try a little of this approach right now.

Clench your right fist and hold it tight for at least 15 seconds. Then say to yourself, "Let go" and, at the same time, let the tension drain from your fist. As the stress fades from your fingers let this continue so that your fist becomes a limp hand, probably hanging downwards. The secret is that, by adding extra tension and then releasing it, we learn a little about the process of relaxing.

The full Jacobson method involves all the limbs as well as the torso and face. What I believe to be important is that you use a phrase of your own choice (such as "let go") and always say this same phrase to yourself as the signal to let the tension drain away. After doing the complete exercise a few times it becomes possible to relax your body at any time simply by sitting down and repeating your personal "mantra".

Talk to Someone

Sometimes we get embarrassed about stress. The reasons for our tensions may be something we have done and now feel ashamed of, a mistake we made, a foolish business deal, a weakness. Even the power of the stress may be so much that we take time to be able to talk about it. Be that as it may, one thing is certain! When times get tough, it's time to talk.

As soon as you can, share your concerns with someone else. This could be a good friend, a partner, neighbour, relative … someone you can trust. If the first person you talk to is not helpful, try another. There are also professionals such as counsellors and chat-lines such as the Samaritans. The advantage of such chat-lines is that they do not know who you are nor do they try to find out. We deal with this theme in more detail in the next chapter.

Get More Information

Dr. Glasser often said that when you do not know what to do, you normally need more information. This happens to me when I go to a new ethnic restaurant. I cannot choose from the menu mainly because I do not understand the terms used. I cannot choose because I lack information. Usually a little help from a waiter lets me know what each item means and it becomes possible for me to make a choice.

Part of the stress experience (and found in both anger and depression as well) is not knowing what to do. Sometimes we even lose the hope of ever finding a solution. Seeking out more information makes a lot of sense in this situation. We might not be very optimistic about making any progress but one thing is certain: if we do nothing, nothing is likely to change.

Plan Your Next Move

Initially when you experience stress you may not be ready to plan anything. However, as soon as you can think in terms of what you are going to do next. Keep it simple, positive and possible. The plan may consist in making a phone call or writing down a list of options. The power to choose is something you do not lose.

Move Forward

All the "emergency strategies" listed in this chapter are mere stop-gaps but have an important function. They enable you to choose something in the short term that will boost your psychological strength enough to take the next step. No amount of deep breathing or relaxation exercises will remove the sources of your stress. Reducing the symptoms does not diminish the cause. It is important that any of the above strategies you adopt (and you might use more than one of them) is only temporary. Eventually you need to turn your attention to finding a solution for your stress.

14. Getting Help

The causes of the frustration that feeds stress can be many. As one comic claimed, reality is the leading cause of stress. The primary solution to stress as outlined in this book is to identify the area or areas of frustration and to take remedial action by getting the information and/or skills necessary to deal with it.

Sometimes it is hard for a person to pinpoint the causes and stress makes problem-solving more difficult since it tends to impede mental clarity. It is very easy to reach the conclusion that there is no solution, that there is no way out. It is vital to anticipate such a thought. It's similar to the thoughts that can accompany a bad dose of influenza; immersed in aches, pains and raised temperatures it can feel as if good health will never return. When you are debilitated in body or mind, hope takes a beating.

What we can do to offset such states of mind is to plan in advance. We need to pre-program our minds with a thought that will rescue us from a position of hopelessness, the thought that sometimes it is important to seek help.

When times get tough, it's time to talk!

This message gains in significance for those in the throes of depression or considering suicide. Talking to someone is vital. Even if the first person you approach does not provide good support, it is important to keep looking. The alternative choice is to do nothing.

The Helper You Need

There are many things you would not discuss with your parents. In fact, there are probably a range of different areas of your life that you would not be keen to share with just anyone. In most cases you want the person to have the following qualities:

- willingness to listen to you
- interest in your point of view
- trying hard to understand you
- not critical or judgmental in any way
- treating your conversation with confidentiality
- honest about the limits of this confidentiality
- knowledgeable about the problem you have
- ideally, qualified as a professional to deal with this problem

People to Talk to

What I recommend right now is that you give some thought to this. Who could you talk to if you found yourself completely stuck in your life? Can you identify one or more people right now who would be top of your list as good people to turn to? When the time of need comes you might not think there is much point in talking but it offers more hope than not talking. That too is an idea worth giving serious thought to right now.

Use the list below to consider the people you know and pick out a few you can store in your head as possible resources when times get tough.

>friends
>partner
>parents
>a teacher
>neighbours
>uncles-aunts
>grandparents
>a police officer
>a social worker
>a religious leader
>a psychotherapist
>a friend of the family
>a telephone helpline
>an online help service
>a guidance counsellor

A word of caution: apart from well-advertised professional help agencies do not open your heart to people you have only met online.

Helping Others

Although this book is mainly addressed to you and any stress you may have, hopefully it will give you an understanding of others together with ideas on how to help them. Avoid telling others that they worry too much or that their problems are not important. Neither is it a good idea to tell them to relax. Instead, listen carefully to what they say, help them identify the problems they have and help them find solutions and make plans.

The Next Step

The next step is yours! You could say that this statement is Choice Theory psychology in a nutshell. William Glasser believes we choose almost everything we do and right now for you that means the next step.

The government might be to blame for the mess you find yourself in. Yes, but the next step is yours. Will you write to them, run a campaign or just go ahead and fix whatever is messed up?

Things might not be going well between yourself and your nearest and dearest. That other person might be blaming you for lots of things or making your life difficult in many ways. Still, the next step is yours. Do you think things have gone too far or will you arrange a chat at a quiet time? Whatever the plan, the next step is yours.

Someone might be able to help with counselling or information. In that case, reaching out to them is the next step, your next step.

That amazing power of choice is in your hands.

Further Reading

Glasser, William. Choice Theory. New York: Harper Collins, 1998.

Glasser, William. Take Charge of Your Life. iUnivers, Inc. Bloomington, 2011.

These books are available in bookshops and libraries but may be obtained from wglasserbooks.com

The Choice Theory in Action Series Titles

A Choice Theory Psychology Guide to Addictions: Ways to Overcome Substance Dependence and Other Compulsive Behaviors - Michael Rice

A Choice Theory Psychology Guide to Anger Management: How to Manage Rage in Your Life - Brian Lennon

A Choice Theory Psychology Guide to Depression: Lift Your Mood - Robert E. Wubbolding, Ph.D.

A Choice Theory Psychology Guide to Happiness: How to Make Yourself Happy - Carleen Glasser

A Choice Theory Psychology Guide to Parenting: The Art of Raising Great Children - Nancy S. Buck Ph.D.

A Choice Theory Psychology Guide to Relationships: How to Get Along with The Important People in Your Life - Kim Olver

A Choice Theory Psychology Guide to Stress: Ways of Managing Stress in Your Life - Brian Lennon

The Choice Theory in Action Series is available from Amazon as e-books or paperbacks and may be obtained through bookshops including wglasserbooks.com

William Glasser International

The body that Dr. Glasser approved to continue teaching and developing his ideas is William Glasser International.

This organisation helps coordinate the work of many member organisations around the world.

WGI recently introduced a six-hour workshop entitled, "Taking Charge of Your Life". This is intended for the general public and provides a good foundation in Choice Theory psychology.

If you are interested in further training in Choice Theory psychology or any of its applications, you are recommended to contact WGI or your nearest member organisation of WGI.

www.wglasserinternational.org

Made in the USA
San Bernardino, CA
27 December 2019

62368241R00075